CHAIR YOGA FOR SENIORS OVER 60

GENTLY BUILD STRENGTH, FLEXIBILITY, ENERGY, &
MENTAL FITNESS IN JUST 2 WEEKS TO IMPROVE YOUR
QUALITY OF LIFE AND GROW OLDER GRACEFULLY

CHAPSHAW PUBLICATIONS

CONTENTS

Introduction   7

1. ANCIENT PRACTICES HELPING MODERN
   LIVES   15
   The History of Yoga   16
   Yoga Is Way More Than Just an Exercise
   Program   19
   Yoga as a Way of Life Today   25
   Exercise: Set Your Values and Goals   28
   Get Clarity and Find Success   29

2. SAFETY FIRST BEFORE YOU START   32
   What Problems Can Limit Your Practice?   33
   I'm Ready! How Do I Start?   40
   Exercise: Know Your Body   42
   Connect the Mind and Body to Keep   43

3. YOGA FOR MIND AND MOOD   45
   Yoga Is More Than Physical   46
   Tap Into the Power of Your Mind   48
   Exercise: Let's Meditate!   54
   A Happy Mind Is a Healthy Mind   55

4. EASE TENSION IN THE HEAD, NECK, AND
   SHOULDERS   57
   What Poses Should I Do to Feel Relief?   59
   Poses for Head, Shoulders, and Neck   60
   Instructions   61
   Exercise: Make Your Own Head, Neck, and
   Shoulders Routine   69
   Keep a Good Head on Your Shoulders   69

5. STRENGTHEN YOUR CORE AND ARMS
   WITH CHAIR YOGA   71
   My Torso and Arms Need Some Help. What
   Should I Do?   74
   Poses for the Torso and Arms   76
   Instructions   78
   Exercise: Make Your Own Arm and Torso
   Routine   98
   Every Part of You Is Connected   99

6. DEVELOP BALANCE AND MOBILITY IN
   THE LEGS AND FEET WITH CHAIR YOGA   101
   Get Insight by Observing Your Body   102
   Poses for Legs and Feet   103
   Instructions   105
   Poses to Help Your Feet   116
   Exercise: Add Your Feet and Legs to Your
   Practice   123
   Keep Grounded   123

7. DEEPEN YOUR PRACTICE WITH YOGA
   MUDRAS   125
   What Is a Yoga Mudra?   126
   Easy Yoga Mudras to Try   129
   The Mudras and Their Benefits   129
   Yoga Mudra Gestures   130
   Exercise: Add Mudras to Your Practice   140
   Gestures, Big or Small, Make a Difference   141

8. OPTIONAL YOGA TOOLS TO HELP YOUR
   PRACTICE   143
   Could Yoga Chairs Be Worth the Investment?   145
   Optional Accessories Are a Helpful Investment   149
   All Tools Are Optional   155

9. YOUR TWO-WEEK YOGA PROGRAM   157
   The Two-Week Program   160
   Instructions   163
   Now You've Started, Keep Going!   181

10. TARGETED YOGA FOR SPECIFIC
    CONDITIONS   182
    Yoga for Knee Pain   183
    Yoga for Back Pain   186
    Post-surgery Yoga   190
    Stroke Recovery Yoga   194
    Yoga for Trauma Recovery and High-Stress   198
    Yoga for High Blood Pressure   202
    Yoga for Joint, Arthritic, or Rheumatic Pain   206
    Yoga for Balance or Inner Ear Problems   209
    Yoga Is Accessible for All   213

    Conclusion   214
    Bonus Audio Meditation   219
    References   222
    About the Author   231

INTRODUCTION

 Aging is an extraordinary process where you become the person you always should have been.

— DAVID BOWIE

Have you ever seen a video of people doing yoga and thought that it wasn't for you? You may have thought, "I'm not the sort of person who can do yoga" and "I definitely can't move my body like that!" You may even have thought that yoga was too offbeat for you.

Whether you have never set foot in a yoga studio and don't know what a downward dog is, or you are a chair yoga expert, you are welcome here. Learning more about chair yoga might be the life-changing experience you need to feel great and move better every day.

There's no question that getting older affects your fatigue and mobility and can worsen your aches and pains. In people aged 65 and older, 49.6% reported that their diagnosed arthritis and pain limited their quality of life (Ferdy, 2004). This means problems with moving as freely as you want and restrictions on what you want to do increase. Even with medical advances, seniors aged 65 to 74 years still experience serious problems in their daily lives with walking, standing, and other daily activities. If you have developed neurological diseases such as Parkinson's or multiple sclerosis, your restrictions may even affect your balance and energy.

Having to get down on the floor to exercise may be out of your current ability range, or you worry about losing your balance and injuring yourself while trying to stay standing. But that doesn't have to be the end of staying active. Chair yoga, an accessible form of yoga practice, allows you to feel supported whether you can walk without help or need to use mobility aids.

Chair yoga adapts yoga poses so that you can safely improve your strength, flexibility, and mobility while elevating your mood so that you feel better about yourself and the world around you. This practice allows those who struggle to stand for long periods of time, suffer from muscle atrophy, or use a wheelchair or walker to feel the benefits of yoga without risking injury. It is also a great practice for anyone who sits for long periods of time at a desk due to a job or volunteering. The chair poses in this book can help you to stay active and flexible while seated.

Chair Yoga Can Change Your Life

You don't need fancy tools: a chair and guidance are all you need. You can use any sturdy chair you have in your home. Now you just need guidance, and that's why you've picked up this book, right? This book is here to guide you along the path of chair yoga so that you can practice effectively within the ability of your body. Even if you have experience with chair yoga, additional insight can help you improve your practice.

So how has chair yoga helped others? Let's talk about Sarah, aged 75.

After Sarah retired from running a business, she felt less able to do what she wanted. A lifetime behind a desk and bringing up a family left her with little time to do more than a quick walk before bed. Her problems with balance and her aching joints bothered her daily. She wanted to play with her grandson or spend time in her garden, but her fear of falling kept her from trying. When a friend mentioned that she had practiced chair yoga to recover from knee surgery, Sarah wondered if it might help her. With her doctor's encouragement, she practiced chair yoga three times a week at home. After a month, she had not only improved her balance, but she found she was sleeping better and was more flexible.

Soon, playing in the park wasn't just for the kids, but for Sarah too.

Many people like Sarah have experienced the benefits of chair yoga. The exercise will get your blood pumping, filling you with energy and developing your stamina. You'll gain awareness of your mind and body, learn how your thoughts can change your mood, and gain control of your breathing so that you can lower blood pressure and stress levels. Changing your physical and mental capacity becomes possible with consistent practice.

How to Use This Book

In Chapter 1, we will set the foundation for your practice: the history of yoga, how you can benefit from ancient wisdom and teaching, and identify your personal motivation to keep you steady in your practice even when your excitement wanes. Next, in Chapter 2, before starting any practices, you will look and see if you have any medical restrictions that will require modifications before you get going. Before moving into *asana* (yoga poses, which you'll learn more about in Chapter 1), we will dive into meditation and mindfulness in Chapter 3 so that you can start a practice to develop your mental fitness and stamina to keep you going through the more physical exercises.

In Chapters 4 through 6, you will find asana for different parts of your body so that you can get started in building strength and flexibility in the areas you need most. Chapter

7 covers *mudras*, an often-forgotten secret ingredient for deepening your practice with focus and mental clarity. If you need more help than a chair, Chapter 8 covers yoga tools that can offer more support, comfort, and deeper stretching.

If you follow any of the practices from Chapters 3 through 7, you will already see a difference in your life within two weeks. For specific guidance to jumpstart your routine, you can follow the two-week plan provided in Chapter 9 that will allow you to get started with a regular practice without having to figure out which postures to choose. As you gain more confidence or desire a change, you can incorporate other poses from Chapters 3 through 7 into your practice. In Chapter 10, you can look further at targeted exercises for specific medical and mental health needs. I will also suggest where else you can find information, exercises, or meditations easily and for free on the internet. These are not required to practice. You have everything you need in this book, but if you want further study, I want to provide you with additional options.

This is not a book that you need to read cover-to-cover, though you can if you want to learn more. If you have never learned the history of yoga before or would like a refresher on the eight limbs of yoga—physical exercise is just one of eight parts of yoga—then reading Chapter 1 will help you have a richer connection to the exercises you are doing and may keep you doing them longer. If you have considerable experience with chair yoga and know that you want to start right away, make sure that you clear your new exercises with your healthcare provider and skim Chapter 2 to make sure that you don't need specific adjustments before you jump straight to Chapters 4 through 6 and Chapter 9 to start the exercises immediately.

Even if you want to roll your eyes at the idea of mental fitness or meditation, I encourage you to read Chapter 3 (meditation and mindfulness) and Chapter 7 (mudras), as you might be surprised at how quickly your mental acuity and resilience can improve by some short, minutes-long practices.

However you read this book—whether selective chapters, a single time through, or again and again—keep an open mind, and you may learn something new each time. If you have read many chair yoga books before, I have a challenge for you: see if you can find something in this book that you either didn't know or that you realize was a helpful reminder. As we all are learning and growing, you are a different person than the last time you took a yoga class or learned about chair yoga. Strive to have a beginner's mind, as if you are hearing information for the first time. You can deepen your practice and learn so much more than you could if you say the dreaded words we all say: "I know that already." Hearing information multiple times in different ways helps integrate it into our minds and lives, and you may learn something brand new to you.

I wrote this book because I know what it's like to have limited mobility and feel frustrated. Often, I wished that my body was different. I also know how profoundly the practice of yoga can change lives, and it doesn't have to involve handstands on a mat. The principles of yoga changed my life and led me to become a teacher, which allowed me the extraordinary opportunity of working with students of all ages. By working with and supporting them as they learn and grow, I watch my students develop a better quality of life. I want that for you, too. Yoga is broader than many of us realize, and it can and should be accessible to everyone. We all start somewhere, and whatever ability you are working with right now, you are welcome here.

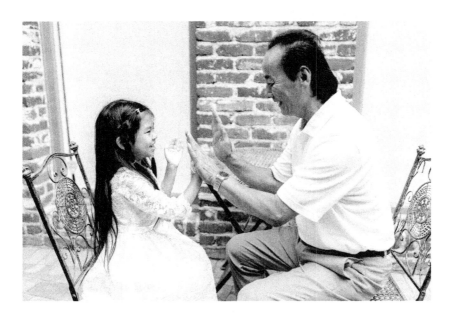

No matter your ability, don't give up on yourself. Try it out to see the difference for yourself. This is about being able to play with your grandkids or neighbors, to have stamina and feel independent and empowered, to have more autonomy and energy, and to have more mental clarity and peace. You will feel inspired, encouraged, lit up, and able to enjoy the years ahead.

1

ANCIENT PRACTICES HELPING MODERN LIVES

True yoga is not about the shape of your body, but the shape of your life. Yoga is not to be performed; yoga is to be lived. Yoga doesn't care about what you have been; yoga cares about the person you are becoming. Yoga is designed for a vast and profound purpose, and for it to be truly called yoga, its essence must be embodied.

— AADIL PALKHIVALA

What do you think of when someone says "yoga?" Do you think of the body as being like a pretzel, bent into shapes and forms?

There's more to yoga than stretching!

There are physical, philosophical, and mental benefits to yoga that, when combined, can make your own yoga journey more meaningful. Learning about the culture and practice can help you make the connection between yoga and a higher state of being.

With yoga's traditions, you can find wisdom that applies to both your chair yoga practice and everyday life. The arms of yoga, its principles and foundation, are as important as learning how to move your body. The more you understand about yoga while respecting its ancient heritage can deepen your connection to your practice. As you develop your mind-body connection, you will have the knowledge that gives your practice purpose and meaning.

THE HISTORY OF YOGA

Developed over 5,000 years ago in Northern India, yoga was first centered in the Indus-Sarasvati civilization. Mentioned in the ancient texts, the *Rig Veda*, the word yoga is found within the mantras, rituals, and songs used by the Brahmans. The Vedic priests used the *Vedas* in their sacred practices. The *Vedas* helped develop yoga as a practice, refining it and creating deeper awareness and connection of mind and body.

Yoga is not a religion and can be practiced by people of all religions, or of no religion, without compromising their beliefs. The original intent of yoga concerned spiritual development to train both body and mind to observe the self and become self-aware. For hundreds of years, yoga was refined by the Rishis and the Brahmans. The *Bhagavad-Gîtâ* is the most esteemed of the Yogic scriptures. Dating back to around 500 B.C.E., the Upanishads created the *Bhagavad-Gîtâ*. The Upanishads internalized the *Vedas'* concept of ritual sacrifice to teach practitioners to sacrifice the ego, letting go of greed and desire through self-awareness, karma, and wisdom (Burgin, 2014).

This practice is demonstrated in three ways:

- self-knowledge
- action (*karma* yoga)
- wisdom (*jnana* yoga)

In Sanskrit, the word *yoga* comes from the root word "yug." There are several translations for this: to attach and hitch horses to a vehicle, to put into active use, or to join. These translations all have similar meanings, though, as yoga is a method of unifying and disciplining the body and spirit.

Yoga is divided into several periods: Pre-Classical, Classical, Post-Classical, and Modern. Modern yoga is what we commonly see about us today, brought to the West in the 19th century by Indian teachers such as Swami Vivekananda and Tirumalai Krishnamacharya and by intellectuals interested in its philosophy. By the 20th century, Hatha Yoga was recognized as a form of physical exercise. Teachers and gurus helped shape modern yoga further through Vinyasa, the flowing transitions between asanas or physical poses. This has led to further forms of yoga being developed and practiced in the West, such as Vinyasa Flow Yoga and Power Vinyasa Yoga.

As yoga became accessible to more people, the need for it to become inclusive led to the use of props and tools. B.K.S. Iyengar helped bring awareness to the need for yoga to be available to everyone, regardless of age or physical ability. His teachings showed props can enable and empower students to continue to perform asanas correctly while reducing the risk of injury. In 1982, Lakshmi Voelker recognized that students with limitations may need more support and developed chair yoga as a form of therapeutic yoga. This yoga style allowed the poses to be achievable and accessible to all levels of physical ability.

For the beginning practitioner, it is important to remember that yoga began with the purpose and desire to bring awareness, regulation, and a higher sense of consciousness to one's being.

How Can Ancient Teachings Help Me?

While it's easy to feel overwhelmed by all the information about a 5,000-year-old practice, it is possible to keep it simple. Learn about how the ancients lived a yogic life, and you will discover the teachings that you would like to bring into yours. In Chapters 3 through 9, you'll discover stretches and exercises to help you achieve physical and mental fitness. You can also enrich your learning by understanding and following the less physical practices of yoga, such as chakras.

To follow this ancient path, keep any or all of these key points in mind while you practice yoga:

- You want to keep your mind and body strong. Your practice can help you keep your body and mind in harmony, improving how you live your life.
- You know you should maintain your body's energy. This can be done through different practices that help you take care of your energy levels and boost your mental health.
- You develop discipline and inner strength. By focusing on building this deeper strength, you can build your resilience in any situation.
- You want to achieve spiritual growth and enlightenment. Yoga's teachings help us realize not only the need for unity and balance within ourselves but the need to connect with and understand the world around us.

YOGA IS WAY MORE THAN JUST AN EXERCISE PROGRAM

While yoga is a great way to develop your strength and flexibility, did you know that movement is only one of the eight limbs of yoga? Each limb is connected to the other, and having them all balanced can improve and enrich your yoga practice.

The eight limbs of yoga, or Ashtanga Yoga, help show this connection. The eight limbs connect from the outer self to the inner self in a sequence. Therefore, doing a posture (asana) needs to be balanced with the other aspects of yoga. Learning the name and meanings behind them will help you understand how connected everything is within yoga and how it can help you connect both with your practice and yourself.

The eight limbs of yoga include the following:

Yama (abstinences): seen as the morals and ethics of yoga. The five Yamas to follow are:

- *Ahimsa* (nonviolence): By avoiding gossip and showing yourself compassion when you need it most, you are practicing non-harming habits.
- *Satya* (truthfulness): Speaking and acting honestly in a thoughtful way means that you practice truth.
- *Asteya* (non-thieving): Neither steal nor desire that which you don't have.
- *Brahmacharya* (continence): Be intentional with your energy and your practice.
- *Aparigraha* (non-covetousness): Avoid being materialistic. Don't worry if you don't have the latest yoga clothing.

Niyama (observances): refers to the positive attributes you should look to achieve. Your observances would be:

- *Shaucha* (cleanliness): Keeping your chair clean and free of clutter.
- *Santosha* (contentment): Every day, acknowledge your accomplishments, such as a pose or a meditation, and feel proud and grateful.
- *Tapas* (self-discipline): Committing to your practice.
- *Svadhyaya* (self-study): You're doing this right now by learning about the history of yoga!
- *Ishvara Pranidhana* (higher consciousness): Realize and feel that you are a part of something bigger than yourself.

Asana (yoga postures): An asana is a posture you hold while staying relaxed and motionless. The pose should allow you to reflect as you remain in the posture and can help improve strength, balance, and flexibility.

Pranayama (breath control): The practice of being aware and in control of your breathing. This can be through deep breaths, timing your breathing, or changing its rhythm. Pranayama decreases feelings of stress, improves mindfulness, and boosts your cognitive function.

Pratyahara (withdrawal of the senses): An act of closing your senses to the outer world so that you may reflect on the inner world. This will help you refrain from dwelling on thoughts concerning the external troubles you may be experiencing, relaxing your autonomic sympathetic nervous system, and boosting your mood.

Dharana (concentration): Often involving mantras, Dharana allows you to focus your mind on a subject or thought without letting your mind wander around. Dharana lets you keep your attention on your practice, avoiding injury and improving your discipline.

Dhyana (meditation): Nonjudgmental and contemplative, you find yourself able to think deeply about what you have focused on, bringing a deep awareness and appreciation. The more you appreciate and are aware of the blessings in your life, and the fulfillment yoga brings you, the more enjoyable your practice becomes.

Samadhi (intense concentration): When it all comes together, you feel a deep connection within yourself and your surroundings. You let the knowledge that you are meditating fade away until it is you, your practice, and the joy you feel. Being truly absorbed in what you practice can deepen your connection, easing any anxiety and bringing peace.

What Other Aspects Are There to Yoga?

Though this book is not about energy work, you may have heard about it.

Chakras are where the energy is centered in your body. Often, they are pictured as whirling disks of energy within the body. These centers can become blocked or overstimulated, leading to symptoms that may be physically or emotionally detrimental to your health.

Asana practices you may need to help any chakra blockage include the following:

- root chakra (*Muladhara*): issues with leg pain (see Chapter 6 for foot and leg asanas)
- sacral chakra (*Swadhisthana*): lack of energy and arthritis pain (see Chapters 4 and 5 for neck, shoulder, arms, and torso asanas, respectively)
- solar plexus chakra (*Manipura*): digestive and liver problems (see Chapter 5 for torso asanas)
- heart chakra (*Anahata*): circulatory or tension problems in the chest (see Chapter 5 for torso asanas)
- throat chakra (*Vishuddha*): may cause throat pain or headaches (see Chapter 4 for head, neck, and shoulders asanas to help this)
- third-eye chakra (*Ajna*): focus or cognition problems, which can be helped by meditation (found in Chapter 3)

- crown chakra (*Sahasrara*): moodiness and lack of sleep (see mindfulness in Chapter 3)

Any of these chakras can experience a block or become either under or overactive. Mentally and emotionally, chakras can affect your creativity, focus, and mood, whether active or blocked. When a chakra is balanced, and the energy is flowing freely, your emotional and physical state becomes balanced.

You can bring balance to chakras through yoga asanas, pranayama, meditation, mantras, and mudras. Practicing yoga can help stimulate your chakras and unlock any areas that are blocked, and you can find chakra-specific sequences and meditations online in videos or courses.

The Bandhas

The bandhas are a practice of locking different areas of your body so that you can manipulate the flow of energy in them. The bandhas activate the throat, abdomen, and pelvis areas. When you contract specific body muscles by holding your breath, you can effectively bind the prana energy to promote energy flow and improve your health. The energy in your body can move more freely inside of you, which brings more vitality to you.

- *Mula Bandha*: the root lock
- *Jalandhara Bandha*: the throat lock

- *Uddiyana Bandha*: lifting of the diaphragm lock
- *Maha Bandha*: all three locks at the same time

Bandhas take considerable amounts of physical and mental control, so they are for more experienced practitioners. If you are watching YouTube videos or reading other books and wondering what a bandha is, now you have some familiarity and you can use it to help advance your own practice.

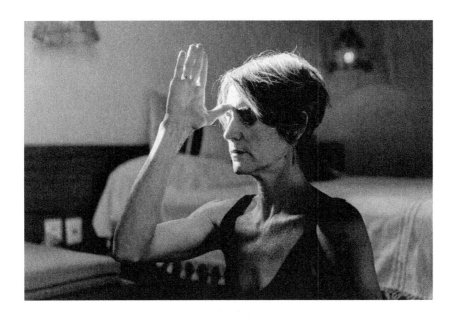

YOGA AS A WAY OF LIFE TODAY

You can practice yoga in the safety and privacy of your own home. You don't need to go to a studio, gym, or luxury retreat. Yoga isn't limited to a daily exercise routine you feel you have to do but can be a part of your life in ways that you may not expect. Learning the ancient names and meanings may seem awkward or irrelevant; after all, your goals are to be strong and flexible! But connecting to yoga on a deeper level can bring more meaning to your practice. That connection will be your guiding star when you need help keeping your practice going.

With a consistent routine, you can feel the benefits of yoga:

- Improve your strength and flexibility, which will improve your balance. With consistency, your breathing and your movements will increase circulation and stamina.
- Decrease your back pain, which is an enormous benefit if you struggle to get through your gardening or daily chores.
- Gain stamina so that you can slowly lengthen your practice time and stay active for longer.
- Ease your arthritis naturally. The pain from arthritis can make it seem like you can never do what you used to do, but yoga can help you change your mindset as you feel relief.
- Maximize your heart health by practicing your breathing and gaining strength. Yoga is excellent at de-stressing your mind, which can help ease the additional stress caused to your heart.
- Feel more relaxed, and that will help you sleep. If you struggle with getting restful sleep, yoga can help

calm your mind and release your thoughts from any ruminating patterns you've developed.

- Experience more energy and less stress! When you feel amazing and energized, and your stress is within your control, the world around you seems brighter. Chasing your grandkids and pets may be a walk in the park after learning to grow your energy.
- Connect with new friends. Yoga is a community, and many people have found lifelong friendships and mentors. No matter who you are or where you come from, yoga has a place for you.
- Love yourself. The little things will add up. What starts as a 10-minute practice can lead to longer practices, more mindful actions, and better awareness of your own health.

Choosing to have the discipline to stay committed to your practice is part of yoga. The Niyama limb refers to your sense of self-discipline and it is a part of yoga that develops with you through consistency.

Having the discipline to stick with yoga can mean that you need to know more about yourself. That self-awareness isn't always easy to unlock, but you're already on that path, and you've started to learn more about yourself. I already know that you are strong and committed, invested in your own improvement because you picked up this book and started reading. Remembering your values when your motivation lags, as it sometimes will, gives you a better chance of sticking with the practice.

EXERCISE: SET YOUR VALUES AND GOALS

On a piece of paper, draw three columns and label them: values, goals, and actionable steps.

Write your values down first. It may take some time to really sort out what matters most to you, but you'll discover them by reflecting on who you are as a person. Examples of values you may have are:

- I am determined and will finish whatever I start.
- I want to be there for my friends, and I'll become healthier and more energetic to make that possible.
- I am taking care of my body and my mind so I can spend more quality time with my family.

In the next column, you can write your goals for yoga. Remember that you can always change them. A goal can be physical, mental, or an action you want to take, and you should tie it to your values.

For example, "I want to go walking with my friends on Saturdays because friendships and my health are important to me. I'll do yoga during the week to strengthen my body and improve my balance" is a goal that ties your value of being a good friend to the goal of walking for your health. Or, "I want to have the energy to have a phone call. I will do the mindfulness practice 5 minutes a day three times a week to build up the stamina to talk freely."

A goal should be something you are excited about, which keeps you motivated to complete it. Your strength, mood, stress, flexibility, and balance can all be improved by sticking with the practice. Follow this value and goal exercise to help you discover the discipline and excitement you need to keep inspired when the initial motivation lags.

When you have written your goal, also write down how you can achieve this. If walking upstairs makes you feel off-balanced and tired, you can decide to practice yoga for 10 minutes two or three times a week to help build stamina and strengthen your muscles. Action steps should always be achievable and small to keep you committed and from feeling overwhelmed.

Once you have your list, keep it in a place where you can look at it daily, like your refrigerator. This reminds you every day why you are practicing, what it means to you, and how you can achieve your goals.

GET CLARITY AND FIND SUCCESS

You may have heard through health magazines or from friends how yoga can improve your life. Now that you understand the history and benefits of yoga, you can commit to your own practice. With an active and consistent practice, you will quickly notice the benefits that it brings to your body and mind. Though at first consistency can feel challenging to maintain, having a clear vision of your values and goals and why you want to stick with this practice will keep you motivated even when it's hard, inconvenient, or even boring.

Sharing the message of yoga means that you should bring this knowledge to others. The act of sharing yoga is a form of self-empowerment, telling others that if you can do it, so can they. You'll soon have done the work yourself, learned the history and principles of yoga, followed a mindfulness and physical practice, and seen the results in your daily life. Not only is that incredible but it is inspiring too.

In the *Bhagavad-Gîtâ*, we learn that we should do things that must be done, tying our actions to the connected awareness of every being (Schware, 2013). Generosity not only helps others but brings you a good feeling, knowing that you have passed on something that can change lives. You have the opportunity to help someone; it doesn't cost you anything, and it only takes two minutes out of your day. You can post a review of this book on Amazon, and you will inspire another senior. With your generosity to share, someone else can learn these tools and decide to get on the path to a stronger body and a more peaceful mind. You help yourself, too, knowing you have helped another person.

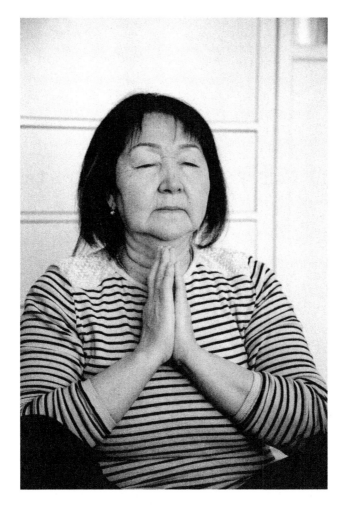

Note: Before you start your yoga practice, check in with a medical professional about what special health needs you have. Consult with your physician about any concerns or limitations you may have.

2

SAFETY FIRST BEFORE YOU START

F irst things first: Be safe. You wouldn't run a 15-mile race if you have never trained for a marathon; the same applies to yoga. Any time you start a new program, you should take some precautions. Chair yoga is gentle and perfect for those who need more accessible exercises but getting your doctor's go-ahead is necessary before you start. This helps keep you safe and reduces the risk of injury. The mental and physical benefits you will get from practicing chair yoga are worth the extra precautions.

Don't push yourself to feel uncomfortable or in pain. As explained in Chapter 1, Ahimsa (non-harming) includes avoiding harming yourself while appreciating and respecting your body for its current state and ability. This helps you avoid yoga contraindication, which is a condition or factor where a particular asana or pranayama can be harmful.

Yoga should be enjoyable! Knowing your limitations ahead of time can be very helpful, but sometimes limitations can arise in the course of your practice. If your body tells you that you need to stop, stop.

The main rule to follow: *If it hurts, don't push it!*

WHAT PROBLEMS CAN LIMIT YOUR PRACTICE?

While you might want to jump right into practice, take some time to really assess your body and your needs. Some common ailments that affect seniors can benefit from yoga but may need adjustments to help that condition in the best way possible. Always listen to your body. Not all of the poses referenced are in this book, but they are good to know as you continue practicing and learning more outside of this book.

Osteoporosis

Commonly known as a bone disease, osteoporosis affects the skeletal structure. The bones become porous and less dense, increasing the risk of breaks or fractures. While this disease is common in seniors, practicing yoga and chair yoga can help create more safety and stability for those with osteoporosis. Since yoga focuses on building muscle and balance, you can help support your structure by strengthening your body's muscles.

Those with a similar condition called osteopenia, where the bone density is low but not as low as osteoporosis, should take similar precautions.

When practicing, refrain from extreme poses. Keep to having a neutral spine, avoiding twisting or bending. You will want to stick to cautious and gentle backbends and mild side bends and twists. During the practice, focus on your movements being slow and steady. Poses that allow you to lengthen the body will help you build flexibility. With chair yoga, you can strengthen your arms and legs without putting too much stress on your hands and wrists.

If you suffer from osteoporosis:

- Do not force yourself into a pose.
- Do not jump or try dynamic weight-bearing exercises.
- Do not perform intense cardiovascular exercises.
- Do not make a quick change of direction.
- Do not practice extreme bends, twists, or forward bends, as this can cause additional stress on your bones. You can still do twists and bends, but they should be mild.
- Do not do any extreme inversions—such as handstands, headstands, etc.—since this will put you at risk for fractures.

What yoga movements you can complete safely and without discomfort depends on the bone density loss you have. Visit your physician and go for a medical assessment and consultation before you start yoga. Slow and steady practice can help build your strength and balance, lowering the risk of injury. If your osteoporosis is advanced and you need to avoid active asanas or postures at this time, you can still experience the benefits of the other yoga limbs and follow the practices described in Chapters 3 and 7 (mindfulness and mudras, respectively).

Sciatica

If you have pain along your sciatic nerve, you likely feel numbness and pain ranging from mild to throbbing or stabbing through your lower back, hips, buttocks, and leg. Typical sciatic problems involve inflammation, tingling or numbness in your leg, and pain, and it can cause you to lose the ability to move easily and decrease your activity levels. You can use yoga to help ease discomfort, but you should still exercise caution to avoid aggravating your pain.

Do:

- stretch hamstrings and glutes carefully.

Avoid:

- forward bends or extreme backbends, which will stress the area.

- poses such as *Paschimottanasana* (seated forward bend), *Hastapadasana* (standing forward bend), or *Kurmasana* (sitting forward bending).

Knee Pain

Knee pain can be from old or new injuries and can be uncomfortable during exercise. By being careful, you can still perform yoga with modifications and careful attention to what your body tells you. See Chapter 10 for targeted yoga poses that you can do while following these guidelines.

Do:

- warm up thoroughly and always practice within your limitations.

Avoid:

- poses like *Trikonasana* (extended triangle pose), *Virabhadrasana* (warrior pose), *Utkatasana* (chair pose), or *Padmasana* (seated lotus pose). They can cause strain on your knees if you are moving beyond your limitations.
- all poses on hands and knees, which can cause too much pressure on your knee joints. This is why chair yoga can be great for your knees!

Hernia and Ulcers

Hernias and ulcers often involve the stomach area, an area many people want to strengthen. Core strengthening is a major aspect of yoga but can aggravate these conditions and cause pain.

Avoid:

- any rigorous core-focused asanas (poses). As tempting as it may be to focus on these asanas for the benefit of strengthening your core, they can cause pain and worsen your condition
- any poses that will compress the abdomen.
- any intensive twists, which will cause the abdomen to restrict and stretch to the point of discomfort.

Hypertension (High Blood Pressure)

A common condition is hypertension, which affects your heart. If you have this condition, you know that additional stress can cause big problems, so try to avoid stressing your body with too much exertion when practicing yoga.

Avoid:

- inversion poses that put additional stress on the heart. These include: downward dog, *Sarvangasana* (shoulder stand), handstand, or *Setu Bandhasana* (bridge position).

Frozen Shoulder

Frozen shoulder is a condition where you lose range of motion, and your shoulder is stiff and sore. You may have even had surgery to fix this ailment. Yoga can help improve frozen shoulders, but you should do all movements slowly and with care.

Do:

- build shoulder strength.
- work to improve your rotator cuff by stabilizing your range of motion and decreasing the pain that often develops.
- keep building your range of motion slowly to avoid damage.

Avoid:

- any poses that stretch the shoulder area and put weight on the joint.
- shoulder openers such as puppy pose, *Gomukhasana* (cow face pose), or downward dog. These can cause pain and stress in the damaged area.

Lower Back Pain

Many people suffer from lower back pain due to injury or chronic repetitive stress. If you are one of them, you should be gentle with your back. You can help by limiting your poses to what feels comfortable and avoiding strain.

Avoid:

- advanced forward or backward bends. These can cause you to overextend your vertebral joints and cause acute inflammation, worsening your pain.

Surgery

If you have undergone surgery or had an accident causing injury, avoid asanas, or postures, for at least three months. This keeps you from aggravating or causing new injuries. When you are able to start or resume your practice, consult your doctor. You will need to understand if and how it may affect your recovery, your surgery, or any injuries you have had. While you are recovering, you can still practice the other limbs of yoga, such as mindfulness and mudras. Read more about post-surgery yoga in Chapter 10.

Post-stroke or Cardiac Problems

Exercise has been proven to help post-stroke or cardiac recovery. According to The Stroke Association, 30 minutes of moderate activity five days a week can reduce your risk of stroke (Exercise and Stroke: How Can Exercise Improve My Health?, 2013). Always speak to your doctor first before performing any exercise. If you are in recovery, you want to proceed carefully to avoid straining your body.

Chair yoga can be a great start, and you should start slowly. Stop immediately if you feel any adverse symptoms or increased heart rate during your practice. If you are interested in learning more, you can find information about post-stroke or cardiac recovery yoga in Chapter 10.

Injuries

Although it can be tempting to try to work through an injury, you should avoid any exercise until you have seen a medical professional. Although yoga is usually safe for post-injury recovery, you should always consult a doctor or physical therapist to avoid any poses that could cause re-injury. Common injuries may include sprains, strains, and tears in your muscles, ligaments, or tendons (Callahan, 2018).

During your practice:

- rest when you need to.
- create stability around the injury.
- adapt your practice as needed to avoid injury.
- stop when you feel pain.

Straining the injury will not help it heal. Be patient and let your body tell you what it needs.

I'M READY! HOW DO I START?

When you are ready to do chair yoga, you're probably excited to start. You should be! You're about to embark on an incredible journey that will improve your health and let you live a full life. But you should know some simple rules to get started, which will keep you safe and injury-free. It will be easy to make chair yoga a part of your life when it feels natural and comfortable.

You will want to wear close-fitting but comfortable clothing. If your clothing is too loose, it can tangle your arms and legs in the chair, which can cause an accident. You don't need to buy clothing specifically for yoga. A T-shirt and a pair of comfy exercise pants are the perfect attire.

The chair you use will be important. You need it to be steady and secure, so it doesn't rock. When possible, choose an armless and straight-backed chair, since your movements will need to be free from restraint. The sides of your chair should be open, provided you do not have balance or inner ear problems. This may not be possible if you are in a wheelchair or otherwise need a chair with arms, but that will not keep you from practicing the majority of poses. Just be sure to lock the wheels of your wheelchair first.

Always warm up properly. This will keep your muscles from injury and lets you ease into your practice. As you progress through your series of moves, keep it slow and avoid rushing. By moving slowly, you can set your intention for each movement. Gradually, you can increase how long you will hold each pose. If you struggle with any postures, especially if they concern your balance, do not move on to more difficult poses until you master the ones that give you trouble.

By avoiding the urge to rush, you will gain more control over your strength and flexibility. Slow and steady will definitely win in your practice. You should enjoy yourself and not feel you need to finish as quickly as possible.

Never push past your limits, no matter how tempting it can be to try something more difficult. You can injure yourself and risk straining your muscles. Always be aware of and acknowledge your limitations. There's no shame in having to take a step back. Your health is more important than proving you can do a hard movement. If you feel dizzy or have the urge to pass out, you need to back off immediately. These are warning signs you cannot ignore.

Note: Always check with a medical professional before you begin a new exercise program such as yoga. If you have concerns or want to know how to address any issues, your physician can advise how to properly take care of your body and how much exercise you can do.

EXERCISE: KNOW YOUR BODY

Knowing all about your body is the best thing you can do before starting yoga. After all, who knows it better than you?

On a piece of paper, make two columns. In the first column, list what concerns you have about your body. These can be current injuries, conditions, or chronic problems that you know you have or are worried about developing.

In the second column, note what poses and types of movements you should avoid, using the above guidelines you've been given. You can also give yourself guidelines about what to do when you feel a certain way. For example, if you know you have pain when you raise your arms, you can write yourself a reminder to not go past a certain extent to avoid injury.

CONNECT THE MIND AND BODY TO KEEP

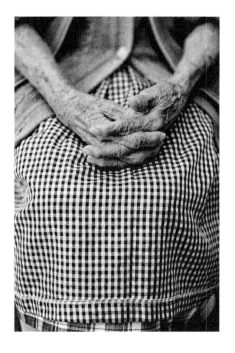

Now that you have done an assessment of your physical health and are aware of the precautions to take, we will learn about one more aspect of yoga before moving into the postures: the mind-body connection. The mind-body connection plays a big part in your entire health system. B.K.S. Iyengar (2019) refers to the body, mind, and spirit being in a state of harmony, and in that harmony, you find health. If your body seems fit and strong, but your mind and mood are suffering from mental health issues such as anxiety or depression, you won't feel your healthiest.

If you feel low or unhappy, it can cause you to avoid your practice and the general well-being of your body. You should treat your mind as well as you treat your body, as they can impact one another. In the next chapter, you will explore how yoga can help improve your mood, let you de-stress, and bring you a sense of peace and joy. Remember to combine the practice of keeping your body and mind healthy jointly, which will let you explore the benefits yoga can bring you.

3

YOGA FOR MIND AND MOOD

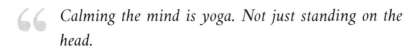 *Calming the mind is yoga. Not just standing on the head.*

— SWAMI SATCHIDANANDA

I f you have been having a rough day and pushed yourself to take a walk outside in the sun, you may have noticed your mind suddenly feeling lighter. Or you sat in the sunshine for five minutes and noticed how your tensions melted away. Afterward, you feel calm and ready to take on any challenges. In that short amount of time, your body has relaxed, and your mind follows that feeling. It distracts itself from any unhappy thoughts by concentrating on the calm state you are in.

You have already learned about the history of yoga and how chair yoga can help your body, but what about your mood? Studies about the effect of yoga on the mind and mood have shown that it can ease depression and reduce stress. One study of yoga participants over the age of 60 reported an increase in both the quality and quantity of their sleep (Brennan, 2021). By increasing the quality and amount of your sleep, your mood gets an instant boost. Over time, this can dramatically improve your life. Have you noticed how much better you feel after a night of good sleep, and how difficult that is to get sometimes? Sometimes a terrible night's sleep can ruin your entire day.

Taking the time and energy to practice mindfulness exercises and improve your mood can change your world for the better. The positive impact of better sleep and a happier, calmer mental state affects not only you but those around you. When you are present with those you love and focused on doing what you love, instead of dwelling on past or current anxieties, you experience life more vibrantly. You'll have more joy in life and bring more joy to others.

YOGA IS MORE THAN PHYSICAL

As you learned in Chapter 1, the poses and physical aspects of yoga are just one limb of yoga. All parts of yoga can improve your life and health. By taking the time to improve your mind and your mood, you can improve your mind-body connection. It may feel inconvenient or even pointless compared to the stretching exercises, but improving the mind and body together will improve your overall quality of life.

Practicing your asanas (poses) properly will help you enter your new yoga lifestyle, and you will learn them throughout this book. Exercising physically can help regulate your mood and bring your body and mind into harmony, and specific sequences can bring about emotional peace and de-stress you. Asanas' ability to help regulate your mood makes them important in your practice.

However, the asanas are only one aspect of yoga you will come to know. If you want to feel the full benefits of yoga, you need to learn about energy, meditation, and mindfulness practices.

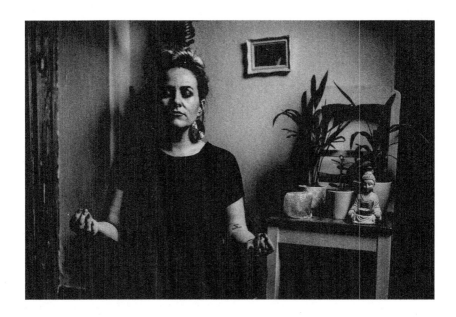

TAP INTO THE POWER OF YOUR MIND

As with your tapas (discipline) for doing exercises, (coming in Chapters 4 through 10), the discipline for mental fitness improves all elements of your health and practice. What is the best way to exercise your mind? There are three proven methods that, when practiced regularly, will increase mental stamina, energy, fitness, and health.

- meditation
- mindfulness
- visualization

These three methods increase your self-awareness and other-awareness, making you a better friend to your loved ones and to yourself. They only take a little bit of time to complete, and you can use them whenever you want to. Your mind, like a small child eating dinner when they want to play instead, may rebel at first and say, "I don't want to!" But if you keep practicing, you will notice the profound effects on your life and may even come to enjoy your daily sessions.

As you grow in your practice, you can start using these techniques throughout the day whenever you need to. You will use your developing skills more often as you grow comfortable with them. If you are waiting in line at the pharmacy, walking in the park, sitting at your desk, or simply sitting at home, you can practice mindfulness.

Meditation

If you have ever been on a vipassana meditation retreat, you know the attendees are called "yogis." Meditation is part of the seventh limb of yoga, dhyana (see Chapter 1). Some fitness classes at gyms are now devoted to meditation only. But you do not have to go anywhere or spend money to meditate. Note that meditation, like yoga, is not a religion and people of all religions can practice. In fact, many religions have meditations as part of services. Medical doctors recommend meditation for its health benefits, which include:

- relieving and managing stress.
- easing any symptoms of mental and physical illness, such as anxiety, pain, or hypertension.
- improving emotional control and health.
- improving memory and cognition.

There are several kinds of meditation such as body scan, breathing, or mantra-based meditations. If you are just starting out, you can keep it simple.

Simple Meditation for Beginners:

- Set a timer for 10 minutes.
- Sit comfortably, preferably in a quiet space.
- Place your hands in your lap.

- Lower your eyes but don't close them completely. You can let your gaze stay on something nearby, such as a wall or piece of furniture.
- Breathe in and out through your nose slowly.
- Focus on how you breathe. Inhale and exhale in a gentle rhythm.
- Begin to count your breaths. If you lose count, start over at one.
- If your mind starts wandering or you are interrupted, simply return to counting your breaths.
- When your 10 minutes are over, take a moment to notice how you feel.
- Repeat daily and add a few minutes every day until you can meditate for at least 30 minutes.

As your meditation practice develops, you'll notice some changes in yourself. By day three, you will feel the difference. Commonly, you will feel a growing sense of peace during and after each meditation, a peace that seems to last for longer periods of time. As your mind relaxes, you'll grow calmer. The focus you gain from meditation will allow your thoughts to not wander as frequently or without your awareness, bringing clarity and sharpness that can help you make better decisions.

You can also explore guided meditations. These give instructions in a soothing way, often with gentle music or nature sounds, and allow you to follow along with the instructor. These can be helpful if you struggle to maintain your awareness and focus. Try Deepak Chopra and Oprah Winfrey's variety of guided meditations, available on chopra.com or YouTube. There are many guided meditations from other practitioners that you may enjoy, and they are available for free on YouTube, Spotify, and online.

While meditation is not an instant fix, your life will change for the better. Be committed to your daily meditation and you will soon notice improvement and find yourself enjoying it as much as you will your asana practice.

Mindfulness

If you've ever noticed yourself lingering on thoughts of the past and feeling upset or unhappy, mindfulness will be beneficial to you. Even if you don't overthink or dwell too much, it can still be something you want to learn. Mindfulness keeps your mind from focusing and ruminating in unhealthy ways. If you think too much about the past or future, it can create a range of intense emotions that have a detrimental, physical effect on the body (see the chakra system in Chapter 1).

Like meditation, mindfulness helps your mind slow down and become aware. Here is a mindfulness practice you can use whenever you need it:

Simple Mindfulness for Beginners:

- Slow down and take slow, deep breaths.

- Bring your awareness to whatever is in front of you right now. This can be an object or thing.
- Every time you feel yourself starting to lose awareness, focus on what is in front of you again.
- Ask "Am I present?" This immediately brings your focus into the present moment.
- Observe your thoughts and feelings as they come but don't dwell on them.

When you are doing chair yoga, focus only on your movements and breathing. Don't linger on any thoughts of the past or future, your problems, or your emotions. By staying focused on your chair yoga, you'll avoid hurting yourself or being too stressed to finish.

A great additional mindfulness technique is to include your senses of sight, touch, sound, smell, and taste. Two exercises you can do easily are mindful eating and mindful listening:

- Mindful eating allows you to fully savor and appreciate your food. Notice each bite of food you put into your mouth: its texture, its flavor, how it feels in your mouth, and how much you enjoy it.
- Mindful listening means you really focus on your companions. You not only listen to what they are saying but how they are saying it, without already trying to form a response in your head before they finish speaking. Their gestures, expressions,

emotions, and choice of words can tell you so much about your friends and family.

To see mindfulness in action and how it can bring peace into your life, I encourage you to read Thich Nhat Hanh's poem "The Good News." The poem reminds us that the good things in life are the special moments and the world around us. We just have to pause, shut out the negativity and noise, and listen. In the Reference section of this book, you can find the book source and a link to the poem. You can also do a Google search to find this poem online. Like he wrote, "you can do this" (Thich Nhat Hanh, 1996).

Being mindful means being present. When you are truly present, you can enjoy the world around you.

Visualization

The human mind is powerful. Athletes use visualization to see themselves winning a basketball game or skating the perfect routine. You, too, can create your own reality with the power of your mind and thoughts.

Follow the simple exercises below to help you craft the perfect visualization:

Visualization for Beginners

- Get clear about what you want. Write out what you want and make it as detailed as possible. This tells your brain to get serious about it.

- When you are visualizing, don't make it just an image. Use all of your senses to see, touch, feel, and smell what you are visualizing.
- Draw it or cut out pictures, pasting those images onto a board. This is a vision board, and it can be as big as you want. Choose images related to your goals and how you want them to look.
- Plan your action steps to figure out how you can get there. This may take some research but that helps you become very clear about what you do and do not want.
- Journal and meditate daily, which allows you to focus on your intentions.

Start with yoga practice. You can use visualization to see yourself fully independent, empowered, feeling safe and confident in your body, and having peace of mind. You can also visualize other goals, in relationships, hobbies, or work.

EXERCISE: LET'S MEDITATE!

If you're ready to start meditating, or you already have some experience, this exercise can help you create a habit of it. It only takes two minutes. You can do this. Just two minutes. By starting small, you're going to build your discipline, and you'll start to notice a difference quickly.

1. Set your timer for two minutes.

2. Take a deep breath and slowly close your eyes when ready to begin.
3. Imagine yourself in a state of calm, peace, and focus. Continue to breathe.
4. Picture what it is like when you are in that state. What do you see, feel, or hear?
5. Notice what your unconscious mind starts to create and the feelings it evokes.
6. Think about how this feeling of calm and peace comes into your life for the following days.
7. Pause and take several deep breaths.
8. Slowly bring your attention back to where you are. Listen to what is around you.
9. Open your eyes.
10. Notice how you feel and reflect on your feelings during the mediation.
11. Repeat this for the next five days.

A HAPPY MIND IS A HEALTHY MIND

We can become so wrapped up in ourselves and what we have going on in our lives that we forget that we have to take care of our bodies and our minds. They are so connected that if you are overwhelmed with stress or anxiety, your body can react with pain or tension, which leads to more stress. You can break this cycle by taking care of both the mind and the body. As you grow older, it becomes very important to take good care of your entire self.

By using these techniques within your yoga practice, you can build cognition, resilience, and happiness. Be patient. Changes in the mind may not happen overnight, but when you stay consistent, you will notice enormous shifts.

Now that you've learned how to take care of your mental well-being, you can start learning to take care of your head and neck areas. These areas can be very prone to stress-related injuries and pain, and you want to treat them with care. If you've noticed yourself having headaches or a sore neck, chair yoga is here to help you ease your pain and help you find relief. Not only is it easy to do, but you'll feel great afterward.

4

EASE TENSION IN THE HEAD, NECK, AND SHOULDERS

Yoga means addition–addition of energy, strength, and beauty to body, mind and soul.

— AMIT RAY

Coping with pain in your head, neck, and shoulders is common for many people of all ages and all professions. This can be especially true if you are seated for long periods during the day, whether because of mobility limitations or due to working at a desk. We carry so much tension that it manifests in these highly sensitive areas. When we hold ourselves with tension, the pain can become chronic. Mindfulness can help ease some of that tension, and adding asanas (physical poses) to your practice can help keep the physical side effects of tension away.

The tension you hold in the upper area of your body from neck and shoulder problems can cause the pain in your head to increase. Irritation and compression of the nerves in the neck or shoulders can trigger pain, which causes a secondary headache. A headache caused by stress or injury can also cause neck and shoulder pain, as can a migraine.

Pain can come from physical, emotional, or chronic reactions. Even simply expecting an awkward conversation can cause increased tension in your neck and shoulders, triggering headaches. If you suffer from temporomandibular joint disorders (TMJ), which affect your jaw and its ligaments, you often will notice headaches and neck pain. Pinched nerves, old injuries, and poor posture also contribute to pain in your upper areas (*What Is Causing My Neck Pain and Headache?*, 2021).

From the time you were a child, you've likely been told to sit up straight and not slouch. Unfortunately, many of us have become used to sitting for long periods of time, whether at the computer working, bent over scrolling on our phones as we look at social media or play Sudoku, or if you are in a chair with limited mobility. You may already feel like your shoulders hunch and that you bring your head and neck too far forward. If you've noticed these issues, the asanas included will help.

Besides your yoga poses for this area of the body, always try to practice good posture when standing or sitting. Your shoulders should keep in a straight line over your hips and your ears should be over the shoulders. It is common for your head to thrust forward if you are using a computer or tablet.

You can also relieve pressure and tension in your shoulders and neck by applying warm compresses, as well as by giving yourself breaks during the day to stretch and relax if you are finding you feel tight in the neck or shoulders. If you have a headache, do your best to avoid any activities that can aggravate it further and practice these stretches to ease any pain triggers.

WHAT POSES SHOULD I DO TO FEEL RELIEF?

Chair yoga for the head, neck, and shoulders is simple and easy. Even if you struggle with stiffness or headaches, you'll notice a big difference with consistent practice. Sometimes your relief may even be quicker than you think.

The poses below can relieve tension in the neck and build strength in your neck and shoulders. This helps relieve both your headaches and back pain while increasing your head and neck mobility. A significant bonus of these poses is that you can do them anywhere, especially whenever you hold your head or neck in an awkward position.

One example of how these poses can help is if you find yourself at an appointment where you are sitting in an uncomfortable chair for a long period. Often your neck and shoulders will ache afterward; take the time after your appointment to give yourself some time to complete these poses. By taking the time to care for your neck and shoulders, you can decrease the likelihood of a headache ruining the rest of your day.

POSES FOR HEAD, SHOULDERS, AND NECK

For the head, neck, and shoulders, learn these asanas to help you relieve tension and stretch these muscles.

- **Neck rolls:** Stretches and release the ligaments in your neck and shoulders.
- **Cow face pose:** Stretches your shoulders and arms, your ankles, hips, thighs, and back.
- **Neck releasing pose:** Relieves any tension held in muscles around the upper shoulders and neck.
- **Chair eagle—Garudasana (for more advanced practitioners):** Creates space and stretches the deltoids and upper back.
- **Triceps shoulder stretch:** Stretches the triceps and shoulders area to open up the chest and back.
- **Shoulder opener:** A flow to open the back and chest.
- **Chair cat:** Releases tension in the entire back and shoulders.

INSTRUCTIONS

Remember the basic rules of chair yoga before you start (as referenced in Chapter 2):

1. Choose a safe, armless chair that is on a secure and flat surface.
2. Keep within your limits.
3. Move slowly and with intention. Stay focused.
4. Keep your spine straight and your posture as good as you can to avoid slouching.

Neck Rolls

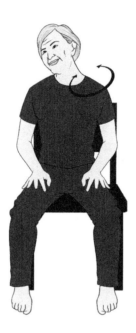

1. Place your hands on your thighs and close your eyes.
2. Drop your right ear to your right shoulder.
3. Keeping your movements slow, roll your head to the center—use your belly button as a guiding point—and continue to roll your head to the left.
4. Breathe as you move your head in gentle circles for five rotations.
5. Change directions and repeat the movement.

Cow Face Pose

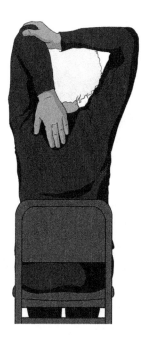

1. Inhale.
2. Exhale and bring your left elbow upward until your arm bends. Your hand may touch your shoulder or back.
3. Pull the left elbow to the right by cupping your right hand over the elbow.
4. Hold this pose for 30 seconds before lowering your hands.
5. Repeat on the other side.

Neck Releasing Pose

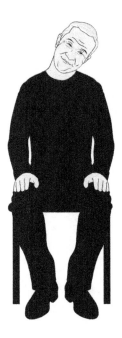

1. Inhale and exhale.
2. Take another deep breath and drop your chin toward your chest.
3. Inhale, lift your chin and head up until you are aligned again.
4. Repeat five times.
5. Exhale and slowly drop your right ear to the right shoulder. Hold for a count of two breaths.
6. Inhale and bring your head back to center.
7. Exhale and drop your left ear to the left shoulder.
8. Repeat five times on each side.

You may notice your shoulders lifting up to your ears. Try to remember to keep your shoulders down as this will increase the stretch and maximize the benefits you will feel.

Chair Eagle—Garudasana (For More Advanced Practitioners)

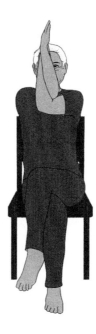

1. Cross your right leg over the left, so that your right thigh is resting on the left. If you are more advanced, you can wrap your right foot around the calf of your left leg.
2. Inhale and bring your arms in front of you.
3. Cross your left arm over the right, nestle your elbows together, and bend them.
4. Touch your palms together.

5. Lift your elbows upward and drop your shoulders down.
6. Hold for three to five breaths before releasing.
7. Repeat by reversing the pose where the left leg crosses the right leg and your right arm rests over your left arm.

If it is too uncomfortable to keep your arms crossed and elevated upright with palms touching, you can reach for your shoulders instead. This gentle hug still allows you to lift your elbows and keep your shoulders down.

Triceps Shoulder Stretch

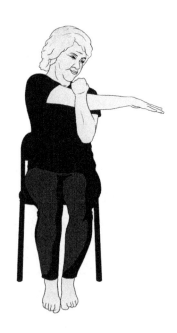

1. Inhale deeply and as you exhale, reaching your left arm across your chest. Your upper arm should be close to level with your collarbones.
2. Lift your right arm and nestle your left arm into the crook of your right elbow.
3. Hold your crossed arm close to your body for a count of 10 breaths.
4. Release slowly and repeat on the opposite side for 10 breaths.
5. Continue stretching both arms, four times on each side.

Shoulder Opener

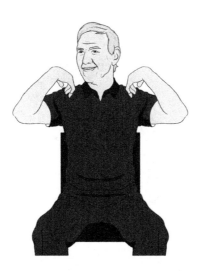

1. Inhale and on the exhale, extend your arms in front of you, keeping your elbows bent.
2. Reach back with your forearms and place your fingers (or fingertips) on your shoulders.
3. Inhale and exhale, opening your elbows to the side while drawing your shoulder blades together.
4. Inhale and bring the elbows forward until they touch. Your shoulder blades should come apart and release.
5. Repeat this for five to ten breaths.

Chair Cat

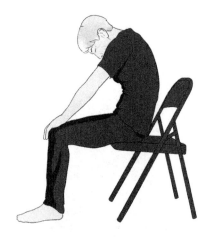

1. Sit with your hands on your thighs.
2. Take a deep breath and arch your back so your chin lifts a bit and your chest is moved outward.
3. Exhale and draw your chin to your chest and allow your spine to round.
4. Hold this pose for two breaths and release.
5. Repeat five to ten times, making sure to follow your inhale and exhale as you move.

EXERCISE: MAKE YOUR OWN HEAD, NECK, AND SHOULDERS ROUTINE

Try each of these poses. You'll probably notice that you like several more than others and that's okay. This shouldn't always be what you find easiest but what feels good and like you are getting the most benefit from.

Write down which poses you enjoy the most. As you create your own yoga routine, incorporate your three favorite poses. You can keep your favorite poses handy so that you can do them during the day as needed to relieve any tension you've noticed in your upper body, neck, and head.

KEEP A GOOD HEAD ON YOUR SHOULDERS

As you build and grow your yoga practice, you'll become more aware of your body. As you practice each pose, you may notice things about yourself that you hadn't before. This could mean that your shoulders feel scrunched toward your ears or that you hollow your back as you sit. Many of the odd positions we mindlessly put our bodies into can create extraordinary stress and pressure on specific areas. The neck and shoulders often experience the first sign of tension getting worse, especially when you feel you are too stiff to move properly.

Now that you have a foundation for improving your head, neck, and shoulders, it is time to look at your torso and arms. Sometimes we don't realize that we need to treat these areas with just as much love as our neck and head. You'll notice a big difference as you work both areas of your body in yoga poses designed to keep you feeling good.

5

STRENGTHEN YOUR CORE AND ARMS WITH CHAIR YOGA

> *At this moment, you are seamlessly flowing with the cosmos. There is no difference between your breathing and the breathing of the rainforest, between your bloodstream and the world's rivers, between your bones and the chalk cliffs of Dover.*

— DEEPAK CHOPRA

Now that you've learned to sit mindfully and to move and stretch your sensitive head, neck, and shoulder area, our focus moves downward. Your arms and torso are connected to your neck and shoulders through an intricate layout of muscles and bones and keeping them all healthy is important. If you are tight in your torso area, it will affect your shoulders and neck because of the way you may compensate with your posture and physicality. Any pain or tension you have in your arms, regardless of where it may be, if the injured area is not cared for, it can cause additional trouble to your shoulders.

The Arms

Many of us use our arms without thought, so often that we sometimes take them for granted. If you have ever experienced a limited range of arm mobility, you'll recognize why they are so important. Many injuries to the arm can result from overuse or misuse, such as tennis elbow, broken wrist, carpal tunnel syndrome, or frozen shoulder. Even something as simple as trying to break a fall can damage the muscle and bone to the point where pain becomes chronic.

Using your arms in yoga isn't just for propping yourself up. They are part of your foundation and can help you find your focus when you use them properly. The arm is composed of several parts: hand, wrist, forearm, and upper arm. Each part can benefit from yoga practice by stretching and developing long and lean muscles. Besides fluid motion and strength, building your arm muscles and bones can help you invigorate your movements and allow you to hold poses for longer periods of time.

The Torso

The torso area is the area that protects your heart and lungs from external damage. Your torso contains the core of who you are. Developing your core (abdominals, pelvic floor, obliques, back, spine, and glutes) lets you improve your balance and flexibility while reducing pain and making movement easier. The other parts of your body that need your torso to feel good are your digestive and reproductive systems, where nutrients and hormones perform major functions to keep the rest of your body going strong.

As the torso, or trunk, holds the most muscles in your body, you'll need to take extra care to avoid any long-term damage or do your best to repair them. Some major muscles you'll be familiar with are your abdominal muscles, which help support your posture and the trapezius which sits on either side of your back, helping you move your shoulders and neck fluidly. There are many more muscles that play an intricate part in keeping your whole body healthy and flexible. When a muscle in your torso is tight or stressed, your range of motion can become limited.

These major components of your health need the right amount of care to be sure they work properly. While you can take care of their internal activity by eating well and managing stress through mindfulness (see Chapter 3), yoga poses can help you build strength and flexibility. Digestive blocks, for example, can be relieved with the right pose, as can any muscle pain in your back. Doing so with attentive care should be part of your yoga routine to keep you moving happily for many years to come.

MY TORSO AND ARMS NEED SOME HELP. WHAT SHOULD I DO?

The asanas (poses) for helping your back, torso, and arm can relieve tension while building strength. You can continue to pick up objects easily, hold things for longer periods of time—like a wriggling grandchild, your sweetheart, or a book that captures your interest—and you can also increase your stamina. Even if you already think you are okay with those movements before starting a yoga practice, these poses can help improve your ability to do them. Instead of grunting and groaning as you move, you will find it easier and less like work—and may stop the groaning altogether!

One of the largest areas for tension to develop is your torso, partly because of the number of muscles and bones involved. Your torso keeps everything together for your vital organs and protects them from harm. Your abdominal region supports your ability to sit up straight with ease while having a strong back and oblique muscles keep you from feeling like you are going to fall over. By practicing yoga, you are letting your torso do what it was designed to do: support and protect you.

Your arms as well are vital to your actions throughout the day. You use them to hug your loved ones, carry groceries, play instruments and make art, and express yourself. Yoga poses can strengthen your arms to make your daily activities easier, creating the lean muscles you need and relieving any tension.

Remember how the poses in Chapter 4 helped you build strength and elasticity in your neck and shoulders, which relieves tension and pain that can radiate to your head? The same goes for your arms and torso. Arm strength can keep you from compensating too much and depending on your shoulder strength to complete tasks. Likewise, taking care of your entire torso can help prevent poor posture and misalignment in your body, such as one shoulder being higher than the other or your core muscles being weak.

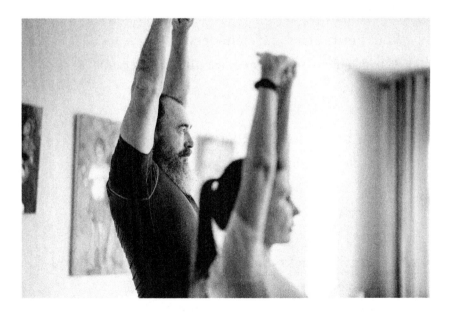

In yoga, it is best to think of your body as a whole, connected unit. With your torso being the largest area that so much depends on and your arms being a major part of your daily functions, you can keep yourself feeling good all over by taking care of these major areas.

POSES FOR THE TORSO AND ARMS

For the torso and arms, you will learn these asanas to help you move and stretch with strength and ease.

- **Chair mountain pose:** Grounds and energizes you before a practice.
- **Chair goddess twist:** Lengthens the spine and twists the torso gently to help digestion and bring energy.
- **Chair arm hold:** Builds stamina and strength for your entire arms and shoulders.
- **Hand, wrist, and elbow rescue:** Releases any tension or pain, stretching your hands and wrists safely.
- **Torso, back, and shoulder flow:** Gives you a full torso and shoulder release and is great if you are seated for any length of time.
- **Chair chest press:** Builds strength and creates energy.
- **Energizing backbend, chest opener:** Opens up your chest and torso, giving your organs space.
- **Spinal stretch:** Relieves back tension and stabilizes your seat.

- **Chair eagle—Garudasana:** Adjusted for the torso, this pose moves your torso and shoulders to open them up and release them.
- **Chair raised hands pose—Urdhva Hastasana:** Stretches the entire body as you reach for the ceiling.
- **Chair cat-cow stretch:** Stretches all the muscles in your torso and back that you carry much of your tension in.
- **Chair side bend (for more advanced practitioners):** Adds length to your sides and releases tightness in your rib cage and obliques.
- **Soothing chair twist (for more advanced practitioners):** A gentle twist that provides a full back release around the lower back.
- **Warrior poses (for more advanced practitioners):** Brings a sense of strength and balance to your body, using your core muscles.

  ○ chair warrior I - Virabhadrasana I
  ○ chair warrior II - Virabhadrasana II
  ○ reverse warrior

- **Downward dog in chair:** creates strong core muscles, lengthens the spine, improves balance, and energizes you.
- **Progressive muscle relaxation for upper body:** Stops you from having an endless cycle of stress and

tension and allows you to notice where you are experiencing discomfort.

———————

INSTRUCTIONS

Remember the basic rules of chair yoga before you start (as referenced in Chapter 2):

1. Choose a safe, armless chair that is on a secure and flat surface.
2. Keep within your limits.
3. Move slowly and with intention. Stay focused.
4. Keep your spine straight and your posture as good as you can to avoid slouching.

Chair Mountain Pose

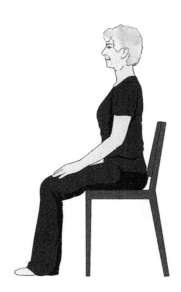

1. Sit slightly forward in the chair. Your feet should be flat on the floor under or slightly in front of your knees. You can use a blanket or block if you can't reach the floor.
2. Inhale and look out across from you as you set your palms on your knees or thighs.
3. Spread your toes and lift your heels slightly. Set them down. Gently rock between lifted heels and lifted toes for several breaths.
4. Inhale and keep still. Feel the ground beneath your feet and the energy in your body as you breathe.
5. Hold three rounds of breathing.

Chair Goddess Twist

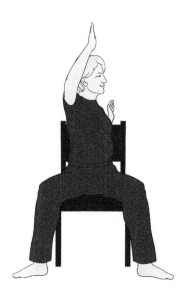

1. From your Mountain Pose, take a deep breath.
2. Widen your legs until they are comfortably spread.
3. Keep your feet flat on the floor.
4. Raise your arms to the sides and bend at the elbows.
5. Inhale as you lengthen your spine and exhale as you twist to the right.
6. Inhale and come back to the center.
7. Exhale and twist left.
8. Continue for two to three rounds.

Chair Arm Hold

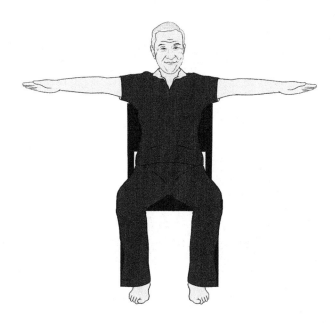

1. Inhale and extend your arms out to the side.
2. Keep your arms at shoulder height as you inhale and exhale three times.
3. Repeat once.

Hand, Wrist, and Elbow Rescue

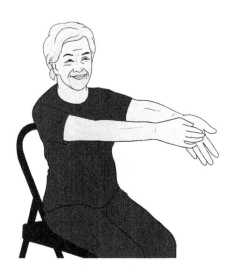

1. Inhale and exhale for three deep breaths. You can keep your eyes open but maintain a soft focus, keeping your jaw relaxed.
2. Lift your hands before your chest and turn your palms toward one another.
3. Touch your fingertips and then move your fingers apart, stretching them gently.
4. Move your palms as if you were pushing them together without flattening your fingers. Imagine you are creating a steeple with your fingers. This will stretch the back of your fingers and the space between them.

5. Breathe slowly and with rhythm. Repeat this pose four times.

6. Bring your right arm forward, palm to the ceiling.

7. Lift your left hand and run your left fingers down your arm to touch your palm.

8. Use your left hand to gently press down your right fingers as if pushing them toward the floor. Avoid pushing too hard; the pressure should allow you to feel a gentle stretch.

9. Repeat on your left arm. You can do this pose several times.

Torso, Back, and Shoulder Flow

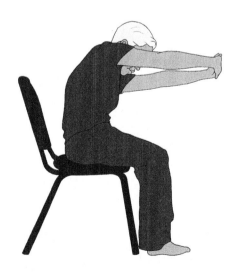

1. Breathing rhythmically, lift your hands from your thighs and interlace your fingers together.
2. Push your palms away from your body as you inhale and let your arms straighten.
3. Keeping your arms elevated, press your palms away from your body in a line parallel to the floor as you stretch your torso forward.
4. Bend gently at the waist as needed.
5. Bring your arms overhead and lift your torso until you are sitting upright.
6. Reach up to the ceiling with your palms facing upward.
7. Exhale. Let your arms come back to your sides.
8. Repeat three to five times.

When you reach your last repetition, you will change your movement:

1. Press upward when your hands are above your head with your fingers still interlaced and palms facing the ceiling. You can imagine you are trying to hold the ceiling up with your palms.
2. Hold for two to four breaths.
3. Exhale and reach your arms forward with your palms facing out.
4. Tuck your chin and round your upper back gently.
5. Move your hands side to side to deepen the stretch in your back and shoulder blades.

6. Hold this for two to four breaths.

Chair Chest Press

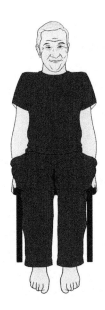

1. Hold the sides of your chair.
2. Inhale and pull up to engage your shoulders and arms.
3. Exhale and release.
4. Inhale and press down into the seat with your hands, keeping your head up and back long.
5. Exhale and release.
6. Repeat two more rounds.

Energizing Backbend, Chest Opener

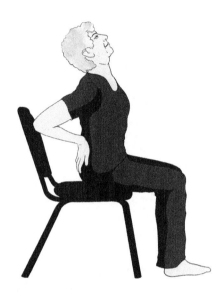

1. With your hands on your hips or lower back, inhale.
2. Look up and continue to inhale. Lift your chest.
3. Gently pull your elbows back to the rear of the chair until your chest expands and your shoulders open.
4. Hold for two to four breaths.
5. Release slowly, allowing your elbows to come back to your sides and your head to lower as you exhale.
6. Allow yourself to relax for two breaths before repeating the pose four times.

Spinal Stretch

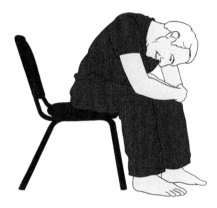

1. Move your feet hip-width apart—approximately 12-18 inches, depending on your comfort level—and inhale.
2. Bring your arms up and fold them over so that you are grasping each elbow with the opposite hand.
3. Exhale. Round your torso and fold gently forward until your forearms rest on your thighs. Continue to let your spine round.
4. Hold the position for two breaths, keeping your head and neck relaxed.
5. Inhale.
6. Pull your belly in toward your spine and roll yourself up, keeping the movement slow.

7. Focus on allowing each vertebra in your back to feel the stretch while rolling upward.
8. Lift your arms as you move until they are overhead.
9. Exhale and allow your arms to return to your lap. Repeat twice more.

Chair Eagle—Garudasana

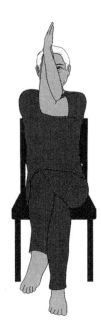

1. Cross your right leg over the left, so that your right thigh is resting on the left. If you are more advanced, you can wrap your right foot around the calf of your left leg.
2. Inhale and bring your arms in front of you.

3. Cross your left arm over the right, nestle your elbows together, and bend them.
4. Touch your palms together.
5. Lift your elbows upward and drop your shoulders down.
6. Hold for three to five breaths before releasing.
7. Repeat by reversing the pose—the left leg crosses the right leg and your right arm rests over your left arm.

If it is too uncomfortable to keep your arms crossed and elevated upright with palms touching, you can reach for your shoulders instead. This gentle hug still allows you to lift your elbows and keep your shoulders down.

Chair Raised Hands Pose—Urdhva Hastasana

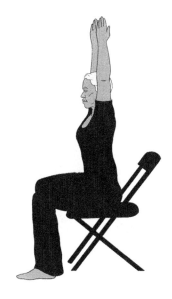

1. Ground yourself in your chair by using your sitting bones.
2. Inhale as you raise your arms toward the ceiling, forming a "U" or "V" shape depending on your ability.
3. Keep your head level and your eyes facing forward, shoulders relaxed.
4. Hold this pose for three to five breaths.
5. Release by exhaling a long, slow breath as you bring your arms down to your sides. Repeat two times.

Chair Cat-Cow Stretch

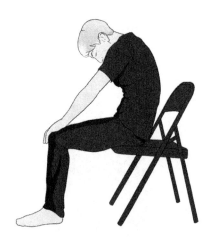

The Cow Position

1. Keep your spine long and as straight as possible as you sit.
2. Ground your feet on the floor and place your hands on your knees or the tops of your thighs.
3. Inhale and arch your spine.
4. Roll your shoulders down and back as you bring your shoulder blades toward one another.

The Cat Position

1. Exhale, releasing the cow position by rounding your spine.
2. Drop your chin to your chest and allow your head and shoulders to come forward.
3. Flow between these two positions slowly. As you inhale, you should be in the cow position. As you exhale, come to the cat position.
4. Follow this flowing movement for five breaths. Release by returning to a neutral spine, relaxing your shoulders, and dropping your hands to your sides.

Chair Side Bend (For More Advanced Practitioners)

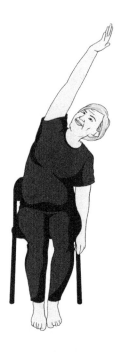

1. Inhale, and keep your right arm at your side as you reach your left arm up to the sky.
2. Continue to allow your arm and chest to lift, feeling your spine lengthen.
3. Exhale as you bend your torso to the right.
4. Hold for two to four breaths.
5. Come back to center and repeat on your other side and practice both sides three times each.

Chair Twist (For More Advanced Practitioners)

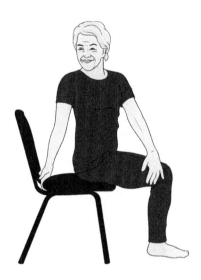

1. Inhale, and bring your arms up to your knees.
2. Exhale slowly and turn your torso to the right, placing your left hand on your right knee and your right hand on the back of the chair.
3. Inhale again and allow your spine to lengthen.
4. Exhale to open your chest and shoulders. Hold this position for two to four breaths.
5. Release slowly and bring yourself back to the middle of the chair.
6. Repeat on the other side and practice on both sides two to three times.

Warrior Poses

Chair Warrior I—Virabhadrasana I (For More Advanced Practitioners)

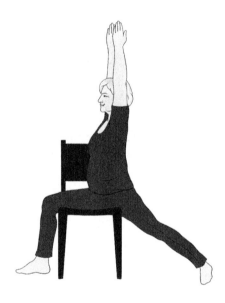

1. Sitting in your chair, slowly turn your body to the right.
2. Move your right leg over the side of the chair and swing or place the left leg behind you on the other side of the chair.
3. Keep the chair below your pelvis and between your legs. Take your left foot and turn it parallel as you firmly plant it on the floor and straighten your left leg.

4. Continue to face over the right side, keeping your hips and torso in alignment.
5. Inhale slowly as you raise your arms to the ceiling. Hold for three breaths.

Chair Warrior II—Virabhadrasana Ii (For More Advanced Practitioners)

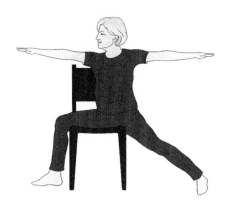

1. Keep grounded as you move out of chair warrior I.
2. Exhale, open your arms and extend your right arm forward and your left arm back.
3. Shift your left hip back so that you can turn your torso to the left. This aligns you to the front of the chair.

4. Direct your eyes over the right fingertips and hold this pose for three breaths.

Reverse Warrior (For More Advanced Practitioners)

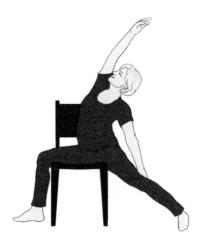

1. Exhale as you release the chair warrior II pose and allow the left arm to rest on the left leg.
2. Raise your right arm to the ceiling as you inhale.
3. Hold for three breaths.
4. Inhale and shift your legs around to face the front.
5. Turn and sit sideways on the chair facing the left. This time, do the whole sequence of chair warrior I to chair warrior II to reverse warrior on your left side.

Downward Dog in Chair

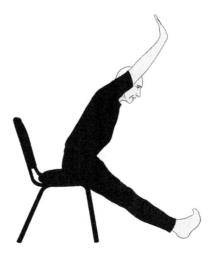

1. Inhale and raise the arms overhead.
2. Exhale and bend forward from the hips.
3. Feel your spine lengthen and hips flex.
4. Hold for several breaths and release. Repeat once more.

Progressive Muscle Relaxation for Upper Body

1. Sit straight but comfortably.
2. Lifting your arms forward, make a fist with both hands.
3. Begin to tighten your arms, shoulders, upper back, chest, jaw, and forehead until you feel tense.

4. Pause for a moment to notice how it feels to be so tight as your muscles contract.

5. Take a long and deep inhale through your nose. Exhale slowly and put your hands on your thighs.

6. Uncurl your fists so that your palms are flat on your lap and spread your fingers. Release the tension in your arms so that they feel like heavy weights hanging from your shoulders. The tension will release in your hands and arms.

7. Allow the tension to release from your other areas: the upper back, the shoulders, and the chest.

8. After you feel them relax, allow your face to soften so that your forehead is no longer tight and your jaw isn't clenched.

9. Repeat this tense and release sequence three times or as much as you need to feel free of tension.

10. When you feel like it has released, observe your body as you breathe to see if there is any tension remaining. Continue until you feel it leave.

EXERCISE: MAKE YOUR OWN ARM AND TORSO ROUTINE

Take your piece of paper with your favorite neck and shoulder poses (Chapter 4) and add poses from this chapter to work on your arms and torso.

In a notebook or on a piece of paper, write down at least three arm and torso poses that you felt helped you the most.

As with your neck and shoulders, you can do these poses throughout your day as needed to relieve tension and improve your mobility. Remember that you can always change your practices as you advance and include or exclude poses as you need to.

EVERY PART OF YOU IS CONNECTED

As you complete the start of a yoga practice by following along with the exercises for your neck, shoulders (Chapter 4), arms, and torso, you will begin to notice how connected everything becomes with yoga. Not only are your body's limbs connected, but within them are many muscles, bones, and ligaments that all share that connection. Remember that along with your body's structure, yoga connects you to your breathing, your emotions, and your mental happiness.

A safe arm and torso yoga routine can give you many benefits, and with chair yoga, you can help create a simple but effective practice. Remember to keep your posture solid and to sit in a grounded position to get the maximum benefits, while remembering to use your core muscles to keep yourself feeling supported. The core muscles within your torso and hips will show the results of consistent practice, with muscles becoming stronger, leaner, and more flexible.

In the next chapter, you will learn about the importance of your legs and feet. If you struggle with walking or keeping your balance, the gentle practice of leg and feet chair yoga can help. As you won't feel the stress and fear of a potential fall, you can focus on strengthening your muscles and improving your balance. Though often the part we forget, the feet do much of our weight bearing and deserve to feel some TLC with some poses that will allow the muscles and tendons to get some relief and a bit of a gentle workout too.

6

DEVELOP BALANCE AND MOBILITY IN THE LEGS AND FEET WITH CHAIR YOGA

> *That's why it's called a practice. We have to practice a practice if it is to be of value.*
>
> — PEACE PILGRIM

Like the old song of "Head, Shoulders, Knees, and Toes" says, the parts of your body affect one another. If your arms and torso are your house, your legs and feet are your foundation. You've learned how mindfulness keeps your mind healthy, and the asanas (postures) you may practice are helping you feel better already. So what about the pillars of your body, the legs and feet?

When you feel a decreased sense of freedom of movement and mobility, your physical health and your mental health can both suffer. A consistent yoga practice targeting all areas of your body can help bring back that sense of freedom and ease. By maintaining a regular practice using your chair, you can develop the strength, flexibility, and balance that can improve your mental, emotional, and physical health.

Taking care of your feet and legs is more than just buying a new pair of shoes that don't make your feet pinch. It takes some time, exercise, and know-how to help strengthen and protect them. Big movements can cause painful tears and ligament injuries, but chair yoga can help you take some weight off your feet so that you can help your lower limbs heal properly.

If you need to use a mobility aid, such as a rollator, walker, or cane, you can practice these leg and feet poses and build up your stamina so that it makes using your mobility aids easier. If you have some mobility but need to use a wheel-chair or sit most of your day, you can use yoga exercises to help avoid pins and needles in your legs or feet.

You don't have to be standing one-legged in an advanced balance pose to experience the benefits of yoga focused on the legs.

GET INSIGHT BY OBSERVING YOUR BODY

Take notice of what your body is telling you right now and jot down what you notice in a notebook. If you are able to stand, you can do a quick self-assessment with a chair for support, but if you need to sit that is fine too. Close your eyes, breathe deeply, and do a body scan from head to toe. Discover the areas of tension, such as muscles that ache or feel tight, any joint pain or inflammation, and any sharper pains. Observe any balance problems or dizziness you may have. Wriggle your toes on the ground to see if you have any pain there. Sometimes we neglect our smaller areas and yet they can be very sensitive.

You can also perform the exercise of *progressive muscle relaxation* from Chapter 5 to discover any areas of tension. Follow the steps provided and focus on your feet and legs to see where there may be problems in your muscles, ligaments, and joints. Notice all areas that may need some attention.

As you go through your leg poses, it can be easy to forget to breathe. Take your breaths slowly and deeply, focusing on keeping your movements as fluid and controlled as possible. Your seat should remain solid on the chair, and you can keep yourself grounded by planting your feet evenly during the poses. If you need to stop and readjust yourself, do so gently to avoid accidentally straining any muscles or tendons.

POSES FOR LEGS AND FEET

For the legs and feet, you will learn these asanas to help strengthen your legs and improve mobility.

Poses for Legs

- **Single leg forward bend—chair Janu Sirsasana:** Improves circulation in your legs and help digestion from the gentle twist at the abdomen.
- **Hamstring stretch—Utthita Hasta Padangustasana (for more advanced practitioners):** Gains easy fluidity to your stride, increasing your confidence in your movement, and less risk of injury as you walk, climb, or play.
- **Chair leg lift:** Helps you strengthen and stretch the muscles which may be tight and in need of release.
- **Chair calf stretch:** Moves and releases any tightness in the calf muscles.
- **Chair boat pose:** Improves focus while working the hamstrings and inner thighs.
- **Chair tree pose with leg to side:** Boosts energy and builds your leg muscles.
- **Chair pigeon pose:** Stretches your glutes while improving balance and circulation.
- **Chair hero's pose—Virasana (more advanced practitioners only):** Releases tight quadricep and hip flexor muscles.
- **Lunge pose using chair (for more advanced practitioners):** Helps improve balance while providing a stretch along your entire leg and hips.
- **Half-splits pose with a chair (for more advanced practitioners):** Improves balance and releases

tension in the entire lower body.

- **Chair extended side angle:** Moves your body to a deeper stretch with a flowing motion.

Poses for the Feet

- **Heel raises:** Strengthens your foot and stretches your heels and toes together.
- **Rolling the feet:** Increases circulation to help reduce numbness.
- **Rocking the feet:** Loosens the muscles in your feet and joints.
- **Loosening and spreading the toes:** Eases any tension in this small area usually neglected by bigger stretches.
- **Ankle circles and flexing:** Increases circulation and loosens the joints and ligaments.

INSTRUCTIONS

Remember the basic rules of chair yoga before you start (as referenced in Chapter 2):

1. Choose a safe, armless chair that is on a secure and flat surface.
2. Keep within your limits.

3. Move slowly and with intention. Stay focused.
4. Keep your spine straight and your posture as good as you can to avoid slouching.

Single Leg Forward Bend—Chair Janu Sirsasana

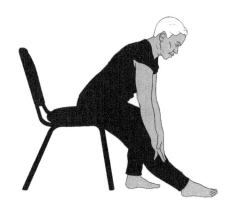

1. Sit at the front of your chair's seat.
2. Inhale deeply as you swing your right leg forward. Keep your left leg bent and your left foot planted on the floor.
3. Rest your right heel on the floor and inhale, lifting your chest and spine toward the ceiling.
4. Exhale, and slowly bend at the waist, chest toward your knees. Go only so far as to feel a stretch in the back of your leg and avoid rounding your back.

5. Hold for three to five breaths and release.
6. As you inhale, tuck your belly toward your spine to sit up.
7. Switch sides.

Should you need some extra help, you can use a bolster beneath your extended foot so that it is lifted or a strap to help you stabilize your pose.

Hamstring Stretch—Utthita Hasta Padangustasana (For More Advanced Practitioners)

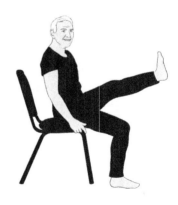

1. Grasp the left side of the chair with your left hand for balance.
2. Push your right leg forward slowly.
3. Lift your leg toward the ceiling, keeping a bend in the knee as needed. Stop when you feel a comfortable stretch.
4. Point and flex your toes.
5. Breathe deeply for three to four rounds.
6. Lower your foot gently to the ground and take several deep breaths.
7. Repeat on the other side when you are ready, using your right hand on the chair for balance.

Chair Leg Lift

1. Inhale and grasp your right thigh with your hands.
2. Exhale as you extend the right leg out from the knee until straight.
3. Flex and point your foot as you breathe.
4. Hold for several breaths.
5. Release and change to the left leg.

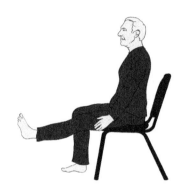

Chair Calf Stretch

1. Inhale. Keep your knees bent as you lift from the ankle, planting your toes on the ground.
2. Lift with the exhale and lower with the inhale.
3. Do several rounds on your right foot.
4. Release and begin lifting the left foot.

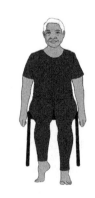

Variation: If you can't reach the floor, place your foot on a block or blanket.

Chair Boat Pose

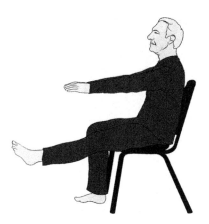

1. Lean back in your chair slightly as you hold the seat with the left hand.
2. Inhale as you extend your right leg in front of you.
3. When you feel comfortable, stretch both arms out in front of you.
4. Hold for several breaths, feeling your abdominal and core muscles engage.
5. Release and switch sides.

Chair Tree Pose with Leg to Side

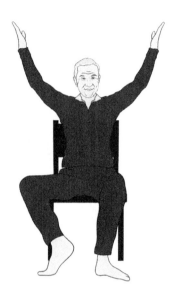

1. Face forward in your chair.
2. Inhale and plant your right foot onto the ground, leaning forward slightly.
3. Bring your left leg out to the side until your knee points outward. Allow your heel to lift so you can balance on your left toes.
4. Inhale. Extend your arms in a "Y" shape overhead or a "U" shape with your elbows bent.
5. Exhale and feel energy coursing through your body. Inhale as you lift through the chest.
6. Take several deep breaths and release.
7. Repeat, switching to your left leg planted and right leg bent to the side.

Chair Pigeon Pose

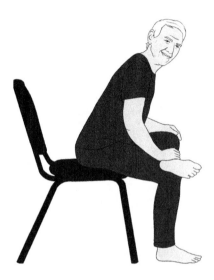

1. Inhale and bring your right leg up toward your chest.
2. Exhale and clasp your knee firmly with your hands and draw your right ankle back to your left thigh. Go only as far as comfortable.
3. Hold this position for five breaths.
4. Release on an exhale and gently place your foot back to the floor.
5. Repeat on the opposite leg.

Variation: If you need to modify this position due to lack of mobility, you can bring your leg up as far as you can. Even when your ankle can only be aligned with your calf muscle, you will still have the benefits of the stretch.

Seated Hero's Pose—Virasana (More Advanced Practitioners Only)

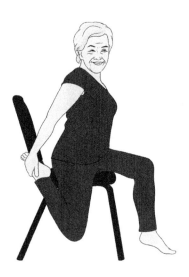

1. Move to the side of your chair until your right leg is no longer braced on the seat. Grasp the other side of the chair with your left hand.
2. Bend your right knee and grasp the foot with your right hand.
3. Lean to the left to increase the stretch.
4. Bring your right heel slowly back and up toward your glutes. You should feel a stretch growing in the top of your right thigh.
5. Hold this position and breathe deeply for five breaths before releasing.
6. Relax before switching to the other side.

Lunge Pose Using Chair (For More Advanced Practitioners)

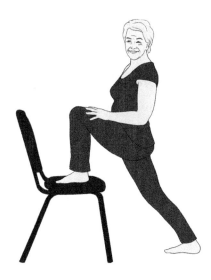

1. Stand up from your chair and turn to face it. You can also turn the chair so you can use the back of it.
2. Position yourself an arm's length away from it, closer if you need to adjust for your own range of motion.
3. Push your weight onto the left leg and foot to ground yourself as you lift your right leg.
4. Place your right foot onto the chair's seat and check your balance.
5. Inhale and as you exhale lean forward toward the back of the chair, so that your right knee is bent forward slightly. You should feel a stretch in your hip flexors and the back of your left calf.

6. Take three to five deep breaths as you hold the stretch.

7. Release and rest before repeating the pose on the other side.

Keep your position correct to avoid injuring your knee by aligning your knee above the ankle and not ahead of your ankle.

Variation: If you struggle with standing, you can sit in your chair. Move until you are on the side of the chair with your right leg still on the seat. Shift your left leg to the rear of the chair until you are in a lunge position but remain supported by the chair. Take three to five breaths and release, resting before you switch to the other side.

Half-Splits Pose With a Chair (For More Advanced Practitioners)

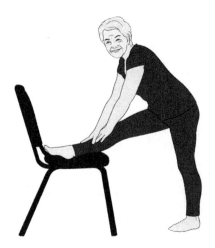

1. Stand before your chair an arms-length away and put your weight on your left leg.
2. Raise your right leg.
3. Lift it until you can rest your heel on the seat.
4. Deepen the pose by slowly moving your hands down your leg as you bend at the waist. You can also stay upright and focus on improving your balance.
5. Hold the pose for three to five breaths. Flex your toes toward your chest.
6. Exhale as you bring yourself upright again.
7. Inhale once more and lower your foot to the floor.
8. Take two deep breaths before repeating this pose on the other side.

Chair Extended Side Angle

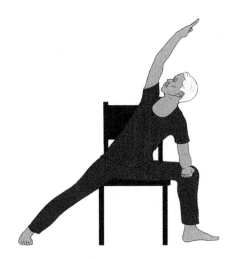

1. Seated, face the front and inhale.
2. Move your legs to form an "L" shape, with your right foot facing the front and your left leg facing outward.
3. Bend yourself until your chest meets your thighs, or however far you can go.
4. Stay in this position as you reach with your left fingertips toward the floor by your foot. If you can touch the floor, great!
5. Inhale again and twist yourself slowly to the right to bring space to your chest.
6. Raise your right arm to the ceiling before bending to the side, as you look straight up to the ceiling.
7. Hold for several deep breaths.
8. Release on an inhale and sit up straight.
9. Repeat on the other side.

Variation: If you struggle with reaching the floor, use blocks under your hand to bring the floor to you. This keeps you from straining your back or feeling off balance.

POSES TO HELP YOUR FEET

If you struggle with your feet feeling achy or numb, yoga can help relieve those sensations and strengthen the tendons. Seniors with mobility problems, diabetes, and circulatory issues can all feel the benefits of yoga. Not only are these stretches simple and require very little strain, but they can be done anytime you need them. Whether in bed, at a desk, or while watching television, you can complete a simple routine to help your feet feel some much-needed relief.

To prepare:

1. Remove your shoes. If you can, take off your socks too. This allows you to feel the full benefit of these stretches while helping you feel grounded to the earth.
2. Sit forward on the seat until the soles of your feet are on the floor. If you can't reach the floor, use a small, raised platform to bring the floor to your feet.
3. Move your feet and knees shoulder-width apart.
4. Keep your spine upright and remember your alignment: the spine should be aligned with the pelvis and head. Do your best not to slouch or allow yourself to tilt.
5. Keep your shoulders relaxed and loose. Your hands should come to rest on your thighs in a relaxed way.

Now that you are ready, try these simple movements to stretch and strengthen your toes and feet.

Heel Raises

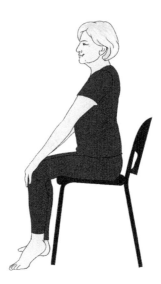

1. Face forward in your chair.
2. Point your toes forward and keep your knees and calves aligned. Avoid letting your legs fall open or become crooked.
3. Continue to inhale and exhale as you begin to alternate lifting your left and right heels. As you lift the heels, keep the ball of your foot on the floor.
4. Continue to alternate your feet for ten lifts on each side.

Rolling the Feet

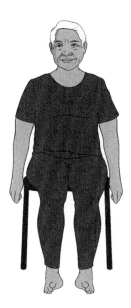

1. Keep your feet shoulder-width apart and plant them on the floor. Keeping your feet on the floor, begin to roll your feet until the inner edges of your big toes and heel are pressed gently to the floor.
2. Roll your feet outward until you are gently pressing your little toes and the sides of your feet to the floor.
3. Roll in and out five to ten times.

Rocking the Feet

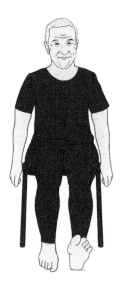

1. Raise your toes on your left foot so that you feel pressure on your heel.
2. Bring your toes down and gently raise the left heel until there is pressure on your toes.
3. Do this multiple times on both feet to create a rocking motion.
4. Repeat five to ten times.

Loosening and Spreading the Toes

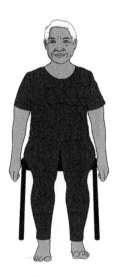

1. Raise your right foot four to six inches off of the ground. Your foot can be lower if that is too high right now.
2. Stretch your toes as far as you can comfortably, wiggling them.
3. Scrunch them up tight before spreading them out again.
4. Stretch your right toes three times and switch to the left foot to repeat the stretch.

Ankle Circles and Flexing

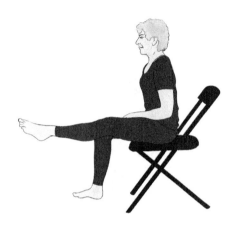

1. Inhale and as you exhale lift your left foot.
2. Inhale slowly as you flex your foot toward you, allowing your toes to point to you.
3. Exhale and point the toes away from you.
4. Repeat three times.
5. Circle your ankle three times clockwise and three times counterclockwise.
6. Lower your foot and repeat with the right foot.

EXERCISE: ADD YOUR FEET AND LEGS TO YOUR PRACTICE

Your yoga notebook is starting to have more poses to practice routinely. Add three leg and foot poses that you can complete comfortably. Try to use poses that give you the most benefit. If you need to give your feet or legs some love during the day, practice while remembering to keep aware of any tension you are feeling. Sometimes the tension we feel during the day is due to a recurring event, such as after a long walk or a specific chore, like washing the dishes. Be aware of these moments and jot them down. You can design your growing practice to help you ease any discomfort or tension.

KEEP GROUNDED

Leg and foot pain can develop from tension in the back, so the back can feel the effects of any issues that you have in your feet. Problem areas in your shoulders may stem from the torso and legs, leading to even more complications. When you no longer feel the freedom of movement and mobility, your mental health can suffer.

Keep developing your yoga practice to include more positions to work different areas of the body. If a certain posture is too uncomfortable or you have been advised against it, you can still use other yoga poses to help build your mobility and strength. With practice, you'll begin to notice differences in your muscle tone and energy levels. Stay consistent and positive. Give yourself lots of compassion to do what feels right and will help you stay active for years to come.

With the body postures now available to you, you can also discover more specialist areas of yoga. In the following chapter, you'll learn about the *yoga mudras*. The yoga mudras are a memorable part of yoga for many observers. These hand movements are motions used to create and improve the flow of energy through the body. This can enhance your yoga practice by deepening your connection and activating acupressure points. Learning the yoga mudras can give you a new perspective on your movements in yoga and a sense of awareness of your body.

7

DEEPEN YOUR PRACTICE WITH YOGA MUDRAS

Yoga is the ultimate practice. It simultaneously stimulates our inner light and quiets our overactive minds. It is both energy and rest. Yin and Yang. We feel the burn and find our bliss.

— ELISE JOAN

You've read about the history of yoga, the eight limbs of yoga, the chakras, the bandhas, and the importance of all parts of the practice (see Chapter 1). As you sit in meditation or move into asanas (physical practice), take it up to another level. Yoga can help bring growth and development, so why not try something extra to build the experience?

If you have seen any representations of yoga in the media, you may have seen familiar images of a seated person with their hands on their lap or in the air. The fingers appear to be in an intricate design or pose of their own. This common image refers to the *yoga mudra*, an ancient practice that improves and channels the flow of energy through your body. Though the hands represent them, the yoga mudras impact the entire yoga experience, from the breath to the emotions you feel. The mudras are a method of communication that many practitioners eventually learn to improve their own practice, as it involves gestures and not words, vital when you want a quiet environment.

Mudras are accessible for anyone able to move their hands. You can practice them in a session or during your everyday activities. The mudras bring a greater sense of peace and clarity to your mind. Though you might be tempted to skip mudras, try to include mudras if you want to experience more harmony and connection with the rest of your yoga practice.

If you want to practice the yoga mudras, you should know the history and the traditions that have kept them a part of yoga for centuries.

WHAT IS A YOGA MUDRA?

Mudras, like all of yoga, are not part of one religion. Though there are different religions that use mudras, it is not inherently religious. Instead, you can find them in many religions and cultures, such as Buddhism, Hinduism, and Christianity, as well as within many art forms such as the Ancient Roman artworks or in the dances performed by Taoist practitioners. Each tradition and religion has a different meaning for mudras; while some may use them for healing, others may use them for prayer. Mudras communicate intent and devotion in ways that words may not, which is important in many religions where praying or meditating in silence may be a sign of faith. However, anyone of any religion, or no religion, can practice the mudras to improve their well-being.

The yoga mudras have continued to be used throughout the years as yoga has spread across the world. In yoga, the mudras can be performed alongside breathing exercises and meditation to improve the awareness and flow of energy that passes through the body. When moving into a pose, a mudra can be used that complements that position and helps the practitioner focus.

Mudras use meridians and acupressure points to activate and cause certain reactions in the mind and body. The act of using these points stimulates your brain. These may seem like simple hand gestures, perhaps not worth learning as much as the full-body postures, but the power of arranging your fingers in this way and activating these pressure points is a lesser-known secret to improving your mental and physical health. The brain powers your nervous system and when a specific area is stimulated, it signals to change the pattern of energy within your body. The brain regulates this prana, or flow of energy, and can influence your mental and physical health.

Your fingers represent the world's elements around you:

- water (*Jal*): little finger
- earth (*Prithvi*): ring finger
- space (*Akash*): middle finger
- air (*Vayu*): index finger
- fire (*Agni*): thumb

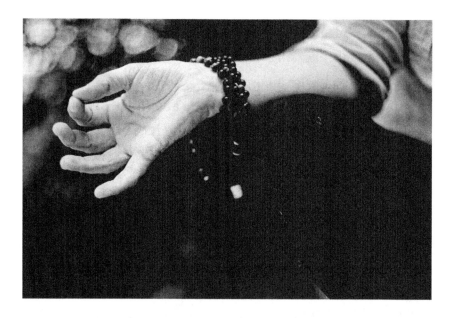

Mudras can seem intricate but are simple to perform with instruction. If you want to improve your mood, attitude, concentration, and alertness, you can add a mudra to your daily practice. While you can do a simple hand position during the day to bring yourself awareness and energy, you can also add them to your asana, pranayama, bandha (see Chapter 1), and visualizations (see Chapter 3) to involve your entire body and mind.

EASY YOGA MUDRAS TO TRY

Remember, refer to this chapter each time you practice to remind yourself of the mudra. The goal is to practice, not to practice perfectly or through memorization. Take as many shortcuts and reminders as you need to ensure a consistent practice. This helpful mini guide will introduce you to the mudras taught to yogis and yoginis across the globe. I will tell you the name, purpose, and how to use your gestures correctly for each mudra. Follow them carefully. As you gain experience, you can experiment with what mudra you need for your mood, mental, and physical health.

THE MUDRAS AND THEIR BENEFITS

- **Jnana-Gyan mudra (psychic gesture of knowledge):** Increases concentration
- **Chinmaya mudra (awareness):** Improves digestion
- **Vayu mudra (air):** Relieves gas
- **Agni mudra (fire):** Increases energy
- **Varun mudra (water):** Reduces tension
- **Prana mudra (life):** Strengthens immune system
- **Shunya mudra (sky):** Brings relief for hearing problems

- **Surya mudra (sun):** Improves metabolism
- **Prithvi mudra (earth):** Grows strength
- **Adi mudra (first gesture):** Increases oxygen to your vital organs

---

YOGA MUDRA GESTURES

Jnana-Gyan Mudra (Psychic Gesture of Knowledge)

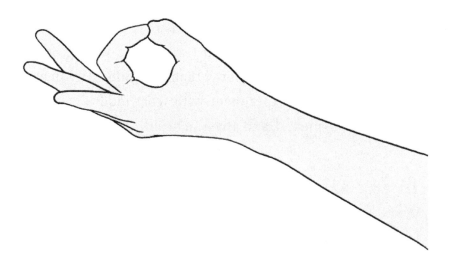

To perform this mudra, your palms should face upward. If you are in your chair, let the back of your hands rest on your thighs. Join the tip of your index fingers against the tip of your thumbs. Your other fingers should be extended away from them.

Known as the mudra for your wisdom and increasing concentration, the Jnana-Gyan mudra may seem familiar if you have seen yoga or meditation in the media. The connection of the thumb and forefingers shows a connection between the higher consciousness (the thumbs) and the individual self (the forefingers). When you make this gesture and turn your palms upward to the sky, you create an open path that connects these two elements. The circle formed by your fingers becomes a seal, allowing energy to flow back into the body in a circuit.

Chinmaya Mudra (Awareness)

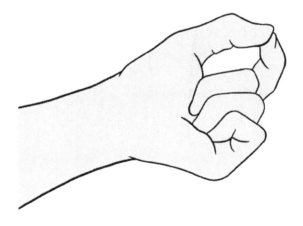

With your palms against your knees or thighs, join the tip of your index fingers to the tip of your thumbs. Your fingers will remain spread gently.

A mudra that can bring a sense of completeness to your meditation, the Chinmaya mudra allows you to feel awareness within your mind and spirit. It may feel or look similar to the Jnana-Gyan mudra but there are differences in the mudras that change their meaning. Chinmaya mudra brings more internal energy, taking your concentration from the outer world and bringing it inward. It brings an increase in energy to your body that flows easier and without any blocks. Physically, it can improve the health of your digestive system.

Vayu Mudra (Air)

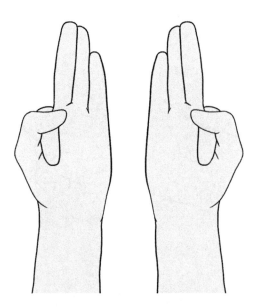

Join your thumb and index finger together while resting your hands on your knees. Allow your palms to face the sky or ceiling to demonstrate your openness and your connection to the universe.

The elements around you are also part of the mudras. The air element is the element of life and breath, and in your gestures, it is represented by the index finger. While symbolizing the nourishing energy that the breath gives us, this air mudra energizes you while connecting you to the world around you, both inner and outer. It represents your mind. This mudra helps relieve the pain and tension in your chest that may be caused by trapped gas.

Achala Agni Mudra (Fire)

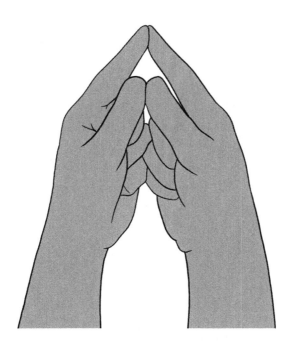

The Achala Agni mudra is performed by interlacing your fingers and pressing your palms together. Lift your thumbs upward to point toward your heart and press them together.

Your hands should rest at the base of your solar plexus, with the thumbs in the upward position. Keep your pelvis and seat grounded as you sit tall and strong. You can look at your thumbs to generate more energy or close your eyes as you meditate.

If you struggle with your weight, digestion, and metabolism, add the Achala Agni mudra to your practice to bring the benefits of this gesture to your practice. Known as a strong element, it is no wonder that this fiery mudra can also make you feel stronger. With its connection to passion and energy, it brings energy to your body and mind. If you want to transform your life and light up your sense of purpose, the Achala Agni mudra can help you.

Varun Mudra (Water)

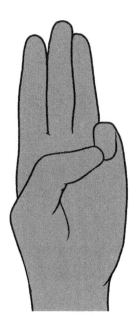

Rest the back of your hands on your knees or thighs. Join your thumb and pinky finger together on both hands to form a circle. Your other fingers can gently spread outward. The pressure of your joined fingers should be soft. If you want to feel more grounded, you can try this mudra with your palms facing downward.

For those who feel blocked in their energy and feelings, stifled by change and tension, the Varun mudra can help you engage and feel like you can "go with the flow" without worry. This small gesture balances you by opening your internal blocks so that your feelings and energy flow more freely in the body. With less resistance, you can move forward in your life and accept change. This water mudra aids in activating the fluid circulation in your body.

Prana Mudra (Life)

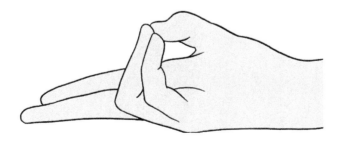

Place the back of your hands on your thighs or hold them in the air. Touch the tips of your thumb, ring finger, and pinkie finger together. Allow the middle and index fingers to touch and extend them outward.

Perfect to give yourself some much-needed vitality and energy, especially when you are tired, the Prana mudra is the mudra that represents life. It strengthens the immune system and helps improve your vision. If you feel a bit low on your energy, engage with the Prana mudra to give you the boost you need.

Shunya Mudra (Sky)

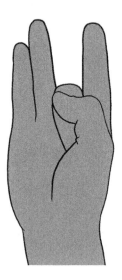

Bend your middle finger and touch the tip of it to the base of your thumb. Cross your thumb over your middle finger and rest it just below the knuckle. You can allow your other fingers to lengthen and point toward the sky.

A mudra that can bring you tranquility and peace, the Shunya Mudra can be added to your meditation practice. You should be relaxed and have a relaxed but strong posture. The Shunya mudra accesses the energy of fire and air to provide relief for hearing and balance problems. If you suffer from motion sickness when traveling, use the Shunya mudra to help you feel grounded and relaxed.

Surya Mudra (Sun)

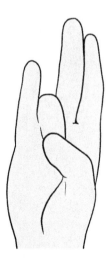

Bend your ring fingers until you can place the tips against the bases of your thumbs. Lay your thumb just above the first knuckle of your ring finger and hold it down gently.

Your other fingers can stay open and lengthened. This gesture allows the fire in your thumbs to increase.

If you often feel anxious and it results in digestion problems, the engaging benefits of Surya mudra will provide relief. The energy that it brings will aid in weight loss by improving your metabolism, which can improve your cholesterol and energy. Associated with the sun and fire, this mudra is great for when you want to boost your vitality. Don't overdo this mudra though; when overdone, it causes too much heat in the body.

Prithvi Mudra (Earth)

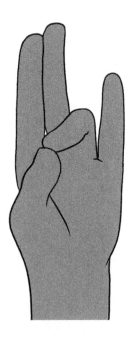

Press the tips of your ring fingers to the tips of your thumbs and allow your other fingers to lengthen and stay straight. This gesture has its best results when sitting in a stable, seated posture.

This diverse mudra has many benefits for practitioners. The Prithvi mudra is of the earth, which means when we are in touch with that element, we feel strong in our bodies and minds. We become stable and confident, able to take on all challenges. Since the earth element is so important to our overall well-being, the results of this mudra are effective throughout the body and mind.

If you are meditating, use this mudra to improve your concentration and tolerance, and to bring patience into your life. If your body needs to gain weight and bone strength, you can also practice this gesture to help you build and repair within. Mentally, you can feel your lethargy start to lessen and your energy improves.

Adi Mudra (First Gesture)

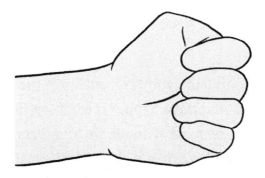

Form a fist by putting your thumb to the base of your pinkie. Fold the other fingers over your thumb. Do this for both hands and place your hands on your knees. Turn your palms upward to increase your connection to the world and beyond.

Called the first gesture because it is similar to the gesture of a fetus within the womb, the Adi mudra brings a sense of calm to your mind and body. By quieting your mind and the nervous system, you can keep anxiety and stress from over-whelming you. When your nervous system is relaxed, you can reduce and prevent snoring as well when oxygen flows to the brain and helps expand the lungs. This increase in oxygen keeps your organs healthy and functioning properly. The Adi mudra brings greater balance and inner connection, perfect for meditation and during a yoga practice.

EXERCISE: ADD MUDRAS TO YOUR PRACTICE

Continue to grow and develop your practice by including mudras. Select three mudras that you believe will give you the most benefit and write them down so that you can remember them. Practice them first to make sure you have the gesture correct.

When you are confident you are making the mudra correctly, start small. Add them to your meditation first. This way you can feel the benefits without worrying about how your asana (poses) may look or if you are getting things just right. As you gain confidence, you can use these with your asanas as well. As you continue to practice these mudras, you can try different ones and note how you feel after each practice. Which mudra you need is not set in stone, and you can use a different mudra as your needs change.

Ideally, practice your mudras with meditation for a few minutes to start. Eventually, you can do your entire meditation with a mudra activated. For the best results, try to do your chosen mudra every day for seven to thirty days. This can be during your meditation, during an asana practice, while walking, or while sitting quietly.

GESTURES, BIG OR SMALL, MAKE A DIFFERENCE

You might have read this chapter title and said to yourself, "This sounds way too weird for me. It probably won't even help me." You could have scanned the benefits and rolled your eyes at the idea that a gesture could affect your entire nervous system or that a fire element ignites passion. It might even have been tempting to say, "I just want the science of yoga, not the esoteric!"

Good. Let's talk about science. Like almost all parts of yoga, science has caught up to the benefits of the practice. For mudras, doctors know that different parts of the brain can be activated by specific small gestures. Dr. Michael Taylor in his work has found that the brain can be activated by small gestures, while the movement of fingers and hands allows for more awareness. By helping reframe the mind and altering your behavior, the use of mudras can change the moods and confidence you feel. The more you use them to help aid your meditation, the more you can access deeper levels of creativity and self-awareness (Taylor, 2015).

Mudras are simple and require less effort than the other areas of yoga. The act of connecting your fingers together in a gesture can bring stability to your whole internal and external self. You don't need any tools or extra instruction to effectively perform a mudra. You can learn and try them at any point in your day to improve your life.

If you think you need some help with making your asanas easier or less stressful to do, you can reach for some helpful tools. In the next chapter, you'll learn about what tools can best help you achieve the maximum results you want while keeping true to your practice and its purpose.

8

OPTIONAL YOGA TOOLS TO HELP YOUR PRACTICE

Yoga begins right where I am—not where I was yesterday or where I long to be.

— LINDA SPARROWE

Whether you are moving your body into an asana (pose) or sitting in meditation, always feel safe and comfortable. Growing frustrated with your yoga practice can cause you to believe that it simply isn't for you and give up before you can really see results. Or, you may have practiced for some time already, but you are experiencing new limitations due to age, illness, or injury.

Yoga is for all people, able to be practiced regardless of age, gender, or body type. The application of yoga principles allows you to find the areas of your body and mind that need some attention comfortably in a way that is non-stressful. You've learned the asanas you need to build a great routine, the mudras to bring you inner and outer connections, and how to develop a safe and simple meditation habit that keeps you aware of your mood, emotions, and physical presence. But what if you feel you need some extra help?

Adding tools to yoga can be a big help if you feel you are struggling. Increasing accessibility to yoga for all people is important, and if you need help, then there is no shame in reaching for a tool to help you. Pushing yourself to power through any problems can cause so much frustration that it can sour your yoga practice and make it less enjoyable.

Using props or buying support tools is not required at all. All you need to do yoga is your chair. However, I wanted you to know that if you feel additional tools would help you, both in going deeper and sticking with your practice, then they are available to you.

Knowing how to appreciate and understand your needs is part of the yoga principles you have learned: do no violence, including to yourself. You should be able to perform asanas gently and with little stress to your mind and body. Tools can help you keep true to that principle.

You can add straps, blocks, beanbags, and massage tools to help improve your practice. By being aware of your body, you can decide for yourself what might be helpful to you. Addressing any past injuries, any illness or disorders, and inexperience is part of knowing which tools would help you. You may also wish to consult with your medical practitioner for any insight they may have.

Remember, there is no age limit on yoga. As you grow older, you are just as capable as any younger person and your own experiences will add more insight into your practice. Acknowledging that you may need some help is nothing to worry about; many younger practitioners use props all the time in various forms of yoga. Being supported by external props is just an extra gift you can give to yourself. It is not required but is often helpful.

COULD YOGA CHAIRS BE WORTH THE INVESTMENT?

Yoga chairs are not like your everyday dining room chairs. While you have been practicing in a standard chair there are chairs that are specifically designed for yoga, especially for advanced practitioners.

Sedentary lifestyles cause enormous difficulties for many people. The harm done to the spine and muscles in the back can cause damage in other areas of the body, such as the nerves or joints. Yoga chairs help correct those problems. Those who struggle with balance and posture may notice a big difference in their asanas (poses) by using these chairs. Instead of growing frustrated and dismayed by the inability to follow a sequence, you can try it in a yoga chair to help support yourself.

There are several types of yoga chairs for different styles of practice. Some of those chairs are: inversion chairs, meditation chairs, backless chairs, and auxiliary chairs. Many seniors find auxiliary chairs great for a gentle practice because of the support they provide, and they can be a good entry choice into yoga chairs. There are more choices out there and you'll need to determine your goals and needs if you decide to purchase a yoga chair.

How to Find the Right Yoga Chair for You

Similar to how you would choose a desk chair, consider your needs.

Do you need:

- a firm flat seat or a padded seat?
- a supportive back or an open back?
- adjustable height or static height?
- something only for one type of yoga?
- foldable or not foldable?
- a solid heavyweight chair or something lighter?
- heavier weight capacity?
- eco-friendly materials?

Choosing a chair made from high-quality materials can improve its lifespan while eliminating any toxins or skin irritants that can come with poor-quality materials. If you have any allergies, keep those in mind as well. High-quality materials can also be eco-friendly, with repurposed metals, wood, and vegan leathers available to craft the perfect chair.

The height of your chair matters. For those on the shorter side, it can be harder to ground yourself during asanas if you can't touch the floor with the soles of your feet. Adjustable heights come with certain chairs, but others will have a static height. Choose the one that will best match your height so that you can put your feet on the ground and feel comfortable.

The seat you need on a yoga chair often depends on what you need for your own comfort. Though a flat and firm seat is great to make your asanas flow smoothly, not every person can enjoy their practice if the seat is too hard. Think about what kind of chair you like to sit on at home when working at a table or desk. You don't want the yoga chair's seat to be cushioned so much that you sink down and can't move properly. If you choose to use a cushioned seat, make sure it is not too deep and the material is waterproof and long-lasting.

The back of your chair will be a matter of preference. Some people may prefer an open back or no back at all, while others will require a firm and supportive back. This can also mean that you would like a longer seat to support your legs. Several chairs come in longer lengths of the seat and back to allow for tall practitioners to feel comfortable. If you're in doubt, see how it feels to sit in your regular dining room chair and take a measurement of its height and seat length, versus your own height and thigh length. You can compare that measurement with many yoga chairs on the market.

Yoga chairs can come in different weights. A heavy-duty chair that is more solid can take more use but will often have to remain in one room only, which is fine if you have an area designated just for yoga. If you need to move the chair around the room or to different areas of your house or apartment, choose something lighter. It also may be helpful to have a lighter chair if you struggle with lifting or carrying heavier objects. Most yoga chairs will have their weight listed so you can take the guesswork out of whether to manage it before you purchase.

Your own weight is also a consideration. Though many chairs can hold a certain amount of weight, it isn't only static movements you have to think about. Moving around on a chair can cause stress on its parts and for the heavier practitioner, it is important to consider what weight a chair can take for the sake of safety. Choose a chair with a maximum weight capacity within your range for optimal performance.

Storage is very important for many people, especially for seniors living in smaller homes or apartments. Yoga chairs that can either be folded up or tucked beneath a table are great for small living areas. Being able to store your chair away means you don't have to worry about making your way around it without bumping and bruising your legs or hips. Lightweight yoga chairs are often very adaptable to different living areas and can be safely stored away after each use. If you have lots of room or don't mind leaving your yoga chair in one space for everyday use, you can consider a chair that doesn't need to be stored away as frequently.

Regardless of its style, make sure that the yoga chair is built with solid components to prevent any collapsing. Choose a chair with rubber feet to prevent any slippage or movement when you don't need it. The durability of a chair is very important, especially if yoga is something you want to take part in frequently.

If you are just starting out, you don't need a yoga chair and can use what you have for now. In the future, if you want to make an investment in a yoga chair, do all the research you can online and by talking to other practitioners. The most important thing to do is just get started with chair yoga, even if your chair isn't perfect.

OPTIONAL ACCESSORIES ARE A HELPFUL INVESTMENT

To help make your practice more enjoyable and easier, there are more options available to help you. Many options are affordable and made with sustainable products that are durable and long-lasting. As with yoga chairs, consider your needs before purchasing, and make any comparisons you need to find a great product.

Yoga Straps Make Poses Achievable

In several asanas, you've learned that you can adjust them by using a looped belt or yoga strap. If you don't have access to yoga straps, you can also use towels, scarves, or a belt. You can use yoga straps during your practice and are comfortable for you to use daily. Even if you are not a beginner, having a yoga strap on hand can help you continue to deepen and improve your asanas.

Yoga straps are made with different materials but a favorite among practitioners are straps made from soft cotton. This material reduces friction and is easy to care for without being too expensive. You can choose to get a buckle on your strap or loops to help adjust them.

There are several benefits to yoga straps that can help your practice. You may struggle to avoid slouching, keeping your leg upright or reaching your ankles. Yoga straps can help you achieve the proper posture and alignment in your body. These straps reduce your chance of injury from straining. By having a yoga strap to connect both hands, or your hand to your leg or foot, you can ease any discomfort while teaching yourself the alignment and slowly deepening a pose.

You can keep using the yoga strap even as you advance to help remind yourself of how a pose should feel, and to relieve any areas locked by tension and tightness. Your yoga strap can help you advance by allowing you to try poses that seemed impossible before.

Support with Blocks

Yoga blocks are simple rectangles commonly made of foam, hard rubber, or cork, and they have many uses. Many practitioners keep them on hand just in case they need additional support. Blocks provide a steady surface, and their rectangular shape is stable.

Having a block or two on hand can allow you to achieve better asanas without worry. In chair yoga you can help relieve tired feet and legs by placing a block on the ground beneath your feet, bringing the ground to you comfortably. You can adapt your forward bends so that you reach for a block standing on its end, allowing you to feel the full benefit of the bend. If you want to extend your arms and your forward bend, a block can be set on the ground for you to reach toward. Even at the end of your yoga session, if you are lying on the ground in the corpse pose (Savasana), you can tuck a block beneath your knees to provide extra support.

You can find affordable blocks in fitness stores or online, including Amazon.

Practice with Pillows

A pillow or bolster can help you improve your practice. Though you can always purchase a pillow or bolster designed for yoga, you can also use one from your own home. Bolsters are great if you are doing any lying down or sitting poses, so they can be very helpful for chair yoga. They maximize the relaxing effect of restorative poses and provide support.

In a forward fold, you can tuck a bolster between your thighs and belly to fold gently over it and rest. This comfortable addition keeps you elevated and helps you avoid the strain that can occur if you are tense and uncomfortable. It can encourage you to open your heart space if you place a bolster down your back and between your shoulder blades. Bolsters can be tucked between your legs or placed on the floor to improve your leg position and bring your feet to a solid surface if you can't quite reach the floor.

Massage Away Tension with Fascia Balls

Struggling with tension and tight spots is a common experience, especially for seniors who may cope with chronic pain or injuries. Self-massage using fascia or massage balls can help when a massage therapist is not available or is outside your price range. The myofascial tissue, or fascia, can cause pain and restricted movement if it is tight or has been injured through repetitive strain.

A common misconception is that for a massage ball to work is that it must hurt before it gets better. But this can be a damaging belief. The harder the ball and the movement you make to get muscles to release, the more likely it is that you will brace and contract your muscles, causing more pain and soreness. Aim for soft rolls and do not dig the ball into your muscles to force a knot to release. Your muscles should feel warm and relaxed, not sore or tense. Avoid several areas as you can damage them: the lower sternum, throat, the tissue connecting your hips and pelvis, the underside of the wrist, the tailbone, and the sciatic nerve area (Hoien, 2020).

Seniors can benefit from this practice by gently rolling the ball over their limbs. Relieving any tightness can allow you to move easier and feel like you can do more, like lifting, carrying, and playing. You can purchase a ball designed for massage or fascia release, or you can use a simple tennis ball to start.

Some simple fascia ball exercises you can do in the comfort of your home, chair, or bed are:

- shoulder massage: Stand against a wall and place the fascia ball under a shoulder. Gently move your upper body in a rocking motion to roll the ball against your shoulder and back muscles.
- forearm massage: Sitting upright, place your bent arm on your thigh so that your palm faces up. With your other hand, gently push the ball with your palm in small circles along your forearm.
- foot massage: Standing or sitting, place the ball on the ground. Place your foot over it and put a little bit of pressure down onto the ball. Roll gently back and forth, from toes to heel.
- hand massage: Set the ball between a flat surface and the base of your thumb. Gently press down on the

back of that hand with your other hand. Move your hand slowly, allowing the ball to roll slowly. Move it up between the connective tissue between your fingers and thumb. To finish, pretend you are kneading bread with your hand and roll the ball. Change to the other hand.

Soothe Exhaustion with Weighted Bean Bags

Any pose that you lie down in, such as Savasana, and reclining meditation can see extra benefits from weighted bean bags used as eye pillows. They place a small amount of weight and pressure against your eye sockets, sinuses, and nose. This pressure can help soothe and relax your eyes. They relax and soften the muscles in areas that we sometimes forget about.

Much like a weighted blanket, the pressure is consistent and not painful. It can feel like a gentle hug for your eye area. The pressure causes you to close your eyes, calming you, and the material blocks out light that may be irritating you and taking you out of your peaceful state. The Vagus nerve is a large nerve in your body that connects your heart, lungs, and digestive tract, and can be stimulated by the weighted bean bags, which improves your mood and calms your heart rate (Mike, 2021).

You do not have to use weighted bean bags or eye pillows only in yoga or meditation. If you struggle with sleep, you can use them to bring calm and relaxation to your body before bed. Though you don't have to purchase one, they can be beneficial if you find relaxing into your meditation or sleep is becoming difficult.

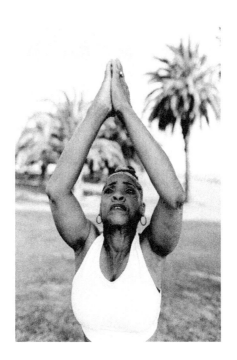

ALL TOOLS ARE OPTIONAL

Yoga tools have been developed to help improve and grow your yoga practice. Their benefits have made them popular with all levels of yoga practitioners and they can help you too if you want to use them. If you think you need the support a tool can give you, give it a try. Experiment with yoga tools if you want to and never feel pressured to believe that using a tool is wrong. Whatever you need to achieve the best results in your yoga can only be decided by you.

Tools are good additions to your practice but in the end, they cannot do the asanas and meditations for you. Now that you have the poses you like and maybe some tools that can help you, it is time to put it all together.

In the next chapter, you'll be walked through a two-week program to help you start your practice on the right foot. This can help if you are worried you might not be able to complete a full practice consistently. Follow along and commit to it for two weeks. You'll see a difference in yourself and learn how easy it is to make yoga a sustainable and enjoyable habit.

9

YOUR TWO-WEEK YOGA PROGRAM

66 *Move your joints every day. You have to find your own tricks. Bury your mind deep in your heart, and watch the body move by itself.*

— SRI DHARMA

Building your yoga practice can be a process of genuine discovery. You'll learn more about your body and mind than you realize. You'll have your ups and downs, days that you forget or days you can't practice because you're swamped, and days where you can't wait to get onto your chair. That's very normal. If you make your practice something you can enjoy and feel the benefits from, it's more likely that you will keep at it.

If you have ever struggled to build an exercise routine, you're not alone. Habits and routines take time and effort. When faced with a decision between what is hard and what is easy, our brains take the easy route. To make yoga practice and meditation a habit, you need to build them into a routine.

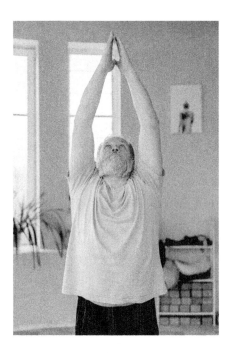

In this two-week program, everything is done for you. You just need to try it. In two weeks, you will notice your body and mind beginning to change. Daily activities and chores will become easier, you'll feel less stress, and you'll even notice some new flexibility, stamina, and strength in your body.

Before You Start

Before you sit in your chair to start, do a bit of reflection first. By getting clear about your intentions, it will be easier to keep going with your practice, even when keeping motivated feels difficult.

- Define why you want to practice: Review your reasons for practicing yoga in the exercise from Chapter 1. Make it personal and you'll find yourself more committed.
- Take on any setbacks: Be flexible with your program if you have a setback. If you have time between a family member visiting and watching the evening news, you can slip a yoga practice in between.
- Take small steps forward: Practice for shorter periods of time to avoid feeling overwhelmed.
- Make the time: Look at your daily routine and decide what the best time could be to practice. It might be in the morning, to help you feel energized, or in the afternoon when you need some extra motivation.
- Be compassionate: Not just to others but to yourself! If you slip up one day and don't practice, remind yourself that's okay. Just move that day's practice to the next day and remember how good you will feel once you complete that day.

THE TWO-WEEK PROGRAM

For this program, you will practice three times a week for 20 minutes each session. If you feel able, you are welcome to exercise more often but try for a goal of three sessions. That will give you six sessions in two weeks, which is a great start. Commit to a 20-minute practice, but if you need to adjust the times for your fitness level, you can.

Begin your daily practice with a warm-up. This gets your muscles feeling warm and loose, reducing the chance of injury.

Move into your asana practice based on the provided sequences. The sequences will target strength, balance, or energy, so you can choose to do one of each for the week.

End with meditation to create relaxation and peace.

Your practice will look like this:

- 3-5-minute warm-up
- 10-minute sequence. Select one of the three sequences provided.
- 5-minute meditation (guided or your own)

The Warm-Up

- hands to heart
- neck rolls

- shoulder circles
- foot to leg flex

Sequence 1: Build Your Strength

- chair mountain pose
- chair chest press
- chair arm hold
- chair goddess twist
- chair leg lift
- chair calf stretch
- chair boat pose
- chair Savasana (corpse pose)

Sequence 2: Improve Your Balance

- chair mountain pose
- chair tree pose with leg to side
- chair eagle—Garudasana pose
- chair twist
- seated lunge
- chair warrior I and II
- chair side bend
- downward dog in chair
- chair savasana (corpse pose)

Sequence 3: Energize Your Body with Sun Salutations

- chair mountain pose
- hands to heart
- chair forward fold and half fold
- seated lunge
- chair cat-cow flow
- seated lunge
- repeat the forward fold
- chair raised hands pose—Urdhva Hastasana
- hands to heart

After each session, you can make a note of how you feel. Compare your first day to the last day at the end of the week to see the progress you've made. Every little step you make is a step forward to feeling great every day and being able to handle any new excitement your life brings you.

Remember to post a review of this book on Amazon to share your experience working with the asanas, meditation, and sticking with a practice. With encouragement such as yours, someone you may never meet might take your words as solace and start a practice to improve their own health. In this way, you are helping to build a community of senior yogis who take charge of their own lives and know they are not alone in their goals of improving physical fitness, mental clarity, and inner calm.

INSTRUCTIONS

Follow the instructions below to build your practice. Each sequence will have a demonstration illustration so you can see how it is done, followed by the list of instructions.

The Warm-Up

This warm-up should be followed before every sequence to help you get your muscles loose and warm, preventing injury.

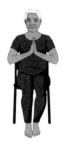 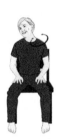 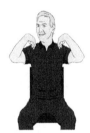 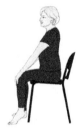

Hands to Heart

1. Inhale and exhale in a steady rhythm as you find your seat. Your back and spine should feel lengthened as you sit as straight as you can comfortably, with your feet on the floor. Close your eyes.
2. Lift your hands into a prayer position and bring them close to the center of your chest. This gesture

lets you feel grounded and compassionate for yourself.

3. Breathe in and out deeply as you close your eyes. Let yourself feel the breath coming into your body, filling your abdomen and lungs with cool energy.

4. Keep breathing in slow inhales and exhales. Take the moment to give the body a scan for tension and pain.

5. Complete six inhales and exhales. Smile. You've started your practice!

Neck Rolls

1. As you inhale, tilt your head back until you feel a comfortable stretch. Exhale.

2. Inhale. Bring your head and neck back to center. Exhale.

3. Inhale. Lower your chin and bring your head down toward your chest. Exhale.

4. Inhale and as you exhale lean your neck to the right shoulder. Hold there for a breath.

5. Bring your head back to center and repeat toward the left shoulder.

6. Keep your breathing rhythmic with the movements. Repeat three times to each shoulder.

Shoulder Opener

1. Place your palms on your shoulders close to your neck.
2. Bend your elbows and press the shoulder blades together.
3. Begin to make little circles with your bent arms. Make two clockwise circles and two counterclockwise circles. Continue to breathe in and out with each circle.

Heel Raises

1. Slowly lift your right heel off the ground. Hold and breathe for two rounds.
2. Place the heel on the ground.
3. Rock your foot back, lifting your toes up.
4. Hold for two rounds.
5. Repeat on the left foot.

Sequence 1: Build Your Strength

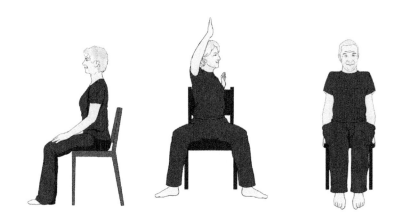

Chair Mountain Pose

1. Sit slightly forward in the chair. Your feet should be flat to the floor under or slightly in front of your knees. You can use a blanket or block if you can't reach the floor.
2. Inhale and look out across from you as you set your palms on your knees or thighs.
3. Spread your toes and lift your heels slightly. Set them down. Gently rock between lifted heels and lifted toes for several breaths.
4. Inhale and keep still. Feel the ground beneath your feet and the energy in your body as you breathe.
5. Hold three rounds of breathing.

Chair Goddess Twist

1. Find mountain pose, and take a deep breath.
2. Widen your legs until they are comfortably spread.
3. Keep your feet flat on the floor.
4. Raise your arms to the sides and bend at the elbows.
5. Inhale as you lengthen your spine and exhale as you twist to the right.
6. Inhale and come back to the center.
7. Exhale and twist left.
8. Continue for two to three rounds.

Chair Chest Press

1. Hold the sides of your chair.
2. Inhale and pull up to engage your shoulders and arms.
3. Exhale and release.
4. Inhale and press down into the seat with your hands, keeping your head up and back long.
5. Exhale and release.
6. Repeat two more rounds.

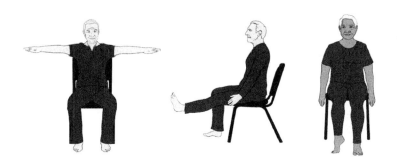

Chair Arm Hold

1. Inhale and extend your arms out to the side.
2. Keep your arms at shoulder height as you inhale and exhale three times.
3. Repeat once.

Chair Leg Lift

1. Inhale and grasp your right thigh with your hands.
2. Exhale as you extend the right leg out from the knee until straight.
3. Flex and point your foot as you breathe.
4. Hold for several breaths.
5. Release and change to the left leg.

Chair Calf Stretch

1. Find mountain pose again and inhale.

2. Keep your knees bent as you lift from the ankle, planting your toes on the ground.
3. Lift with the exhale and lower with the inhale.
4. Do several rounds on your right foot.
5. Release and begin lifting the left foot.

Variation: If you can't reach the floor, place your foot on a block or blanket.

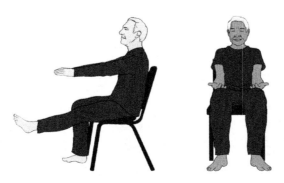

Chair Boat Pose

1. Lean back in your chair slightly as you hold the seat with your left hand.
2. Inhale as you extend your right leg in front of you.
3. When you feel comfortable, stretch both arms out in front of you.
4. Hold for several breaths, feeling your abdominal and core muscles engage.
5. Release and switch sides.

Chair Savasana (Corpse Pose)

1. In your chair, sit with your eyes closed and your hands resting loosely in your lap.
2. Let your spine remain long and the shoulders back.
3. Observe any sensations in your body.
4. Start with 12 rounds of breathing. You can sit in Savasana for as long as needed.

Sequence 2: Improve Your Balance

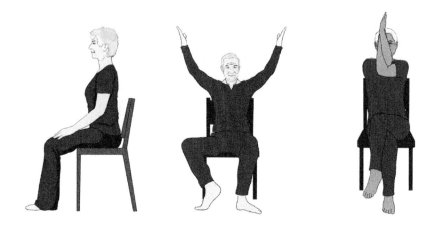

Chair Mountain Pose

1. Sit slightly forward in the chair. Your feet should be flat on the floor under or slightly in front of your knees. You can use a blanket or block if you can't reach the floor.

2. Inhale and look out across from you as you set your palms on your knees or thighs.
3. Spread your toes and lift your heels slightly. Set them down. Gently rock between lifted heels and lifted toes for several breaths.
4. Inhale and keep still. Feel the ground beneath your feet and the energy in your body as you breathe.
5. Hold three rounds of breathing.

Chair Tree Pose with Leg to Side

1. Face forward in your chair.
2. Inhale and plant your right foot onto the ground, leaning forward slightly.
3. Bring your left leg out to the side until your knee points outward. Allow your heel to lift so you can balance on your left toes.
4. Inhale. Extend your arms in a "Y" shape overhead or a "U" shape with your elbows bent.
5. Exhale and feel energy coursing through your body. Inhale as you lift through the chest.
6. Take several deep breaths and release.
7. Repeat, switching to your left leg planted and right leg bent to the side.

Chair Eagle—Garudasana Pose

1. Cross your right leg over your left.

2. Bend your right arm and place your left arm beneath it, holding your right elbow.

3. Reach up with the left hand to try to place the back of your hands against each other.

4. Inhale as you gently lift your elbows and shoulders. Exhale to bring them down.

5. Repeat for three breaths and switch to the other side (right arm below left arm and left leg over your right).

Variations: You can cross your ankles if crossing your legs is too difficult. If you struggle to bend and lift your arms, take each hand to the opposite shoulder and give yourself a gentle hug.

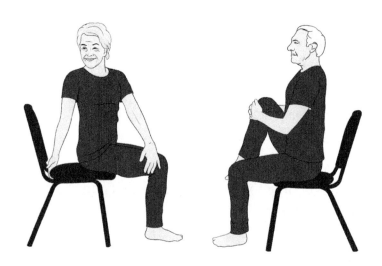

Chair Twist

1. Grasp your chair's sides with each hand.
2. Inhale. Turn your torso slowly to the right, letting it twist from the hip area. Your hips and core muscles will be engaged.
3. Look behind yourself and exhale.
4. Take one breath, in and out.
5. Inhale again as you come back to the center. Complete this movement to the right twice more.
6. Repeat to the left.

Seated Lunge

1. Inhale. Lift your right leg up, supporting with your hands beneath your thigh.
2. Raise your right thigh toward your chest, bending at the knee.
3. Hold for two to three breaths.
4. Release and switch legs.
5. Repeat once more.

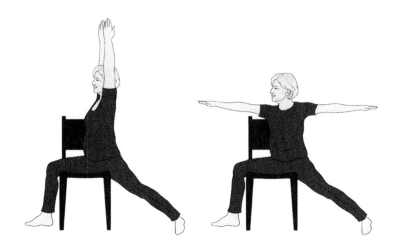

Chair Warrior I and II

1. Inhale as you bring your left foot out to the side, pointing your toes out with your knee bent.
2. Extend your right foot behind you to the right of your chair.
3. Exhale and bring your arms up to shoulder level. Look out over your left hand.
4. Inhale and exhale deeply, holding for three breaths.
5. Inhale to release and return to center.
6. Repeat on the other side, bending your right knee and extending the left leg behind. Hold for three breaths.

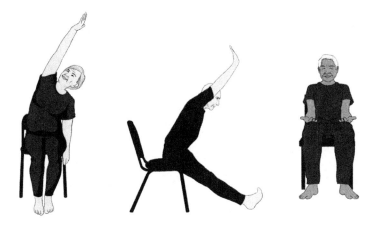

Chair Side Bend

1. Sit back in a neutral spine, centered and calm. Keep your shoulders rolled back and chest open.
2. As you lift your right fingers up to the sky (palm in), place your left fingertips on the floor. Stretch through the right side of your body as you slowly bend to the left.
3. Keep your right shoulder down and your seat grounded as you stretch from hip to fingertips.
4. Hold for five breaths and return to center.
5. Repeat to stretch the left side.

Downward Dog in Chair

1. Begin in mountain pose.
2. Inhale and raise the arms overhead.
3. Exhale and bend forward from the hips.

4. Feel your spine lengthen and hips flex.

5. Hold for several breaths and release. Repeat once more.

Chair Savasana

Repeat as in Sequence 1

Sequence 3: Energize Your Body with Sun Salutations

Sun salutations are great for a warm-up but also can energize and help you gain confidence with chair yoga.

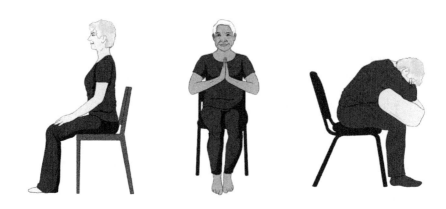

Chair Mountain Pose

1. Sit slightly forward in the chair. Your feet should be flat on the floor under or slightly in front of your knees. You can use a blanket or block if you can't reach the floor.

2. Inhale and look out across from you as you set your palms on your knees or thighs.

3. Spread your toes and lift your heels slightly. Set them down. Gently rock between lifted heels and lifted toes for several breaths.

4. Inhale and keep still. Feel the ground beneath your feet and the energy in your body as you breathe.

5. Hold three rounds of breathing.

Hands to Heart

1. Exhale and bring your palms to prayer position in front of your chest.

2. Inhale and lift your arms slowly to the front, stretching them upward to the ceiling. Take your gaze up past your hands.

Chair Forward Fold and Half Fold

1. Exhale. Take your hands from their extended backward pose and bend gently forward.

2. Bend at your torso as you exhale and let your arms come to your legs. Your hands can fall to your knees, shins, or feet, depending on your ability and comfort.

3. Rest your torso on your thighs and place your chin close to your knees as you stare at the ground.

4. Breathe in and out. Let your torso fall closer to the thighs and stretch your shoulders. If you can, place your hand on the floor or on your lower leg.

5. Remain for two to four breaths.

6. Inhale and lift your torso halfway until your body forms an angle.

7. Hold for one breath and exhale as you fold toward your knees again.

8. Release and rise to sitting upright again.

Variation: Place a bolster or pillow on your thighs to make the forward fold easier as you rest your torso on the bolster.

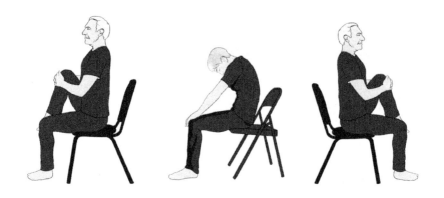

Seated Lunge—Right

1. Inhale and take your right thigh in your hands.

2. Lift the thigh toward your belly as you look ahead.

3. Release as you exhale to put your foot back on the ground.

Chair Cat-Cow Flow

1. Inhale and put your hands on your knees.
2. Let your shoulders roll back as your chest comes out.
3. Drop your head back as you maintain a long back.
4. Exhale as you curl your spine and tuck your chin down to the chest. Roll back gently on your tailbone.
5. Repeat for three breaths, flowing between cow and cat poses.

Seated Lunge—Left

1. Inhale and take your left thigh in your hands.
2. Lift the thigh toward your belly as you look ahead.
3. Release as you exhale to put your foot back on the ground.

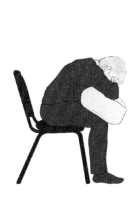
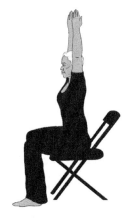
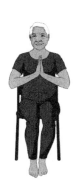

Repeat the Forward Fold

Chair Raised Hands Pose—Urdhva Hastasana

1. Inhale and place your hands on your thighs.
2. Exhale as you lift your arms to the sky, following the movement with your eyes until your chin lifts.
3. Hold for three breaths before putting your arms down and sitting up straight.

Hands to Heart

1. Exhale and bring your palms to the prayer position in front of your chest.

Post-Workout Meditation

After each asana session, take the time to spend at least 5 minutes in guided meditation. You can find great ones on Spotify, Apple, YouTube, or other online resources.

If you want to do your own mediation, set a timer for 5 minutes.

The 5 minutes of meditation can help you reflect on your time in the chair and give your mind time to relax and process what your body feels.

NOW YOU'VE STARTED, KEEP GOING!

This program allows you to experience different poses that help strengthen your body and bring you balance and energy. By committing to 2 weeks, you can start building a lasting habit. You can refer to these exercises to create your own sequence. If a pose feels too difficult or stressful, try a modification with a strap or pillow. You can also change that pose for something you find more achievable.

Do you have a condition that you feel could limit your practice? Yoga can be adapted to many types of medical conditions and needs. Now that you've learned how a sequence can bring you strength and balance, you will learn how certain asanas can help you adapt your practice to your needs.

10

TARGETED YOGA FOR SPECIFIC CONDITIONS

The yoga pose is not the goal. Becoming flexible is not the goal. Standing on your hands is not the goal. The goal is serenity. Balance. Truly finding peace in your own skin.

— RACHEL BRATHEN

When you've read the history of yoga, followed the mindfulness practices, tried a mudra or two, and tried the asanas (postures), you may still have some hesitation. Several medical conditions, whether from illness or injury, can make some things seem less achievable. You still want the benefits of yoga, but you're worried you could harm your body.

You can do the other seven limbs of yoga, but you really would love to try some asanas that cater to your specific needs. With your doctor's guidance, you can try asanas, while still listening to your body and its abilities. The options below can be very helpful for you to experience the benefits of yoga, adapted for you to keep the practices simple and targeted to help improve your body.

Before starting any new exercise routine, always consult your doctor. They may have additional resources and guidelines for you to follow to make sure you can practice safely.

YOGA FOR KNEE PAIN

Knee pain is a common complaint for all ages, but it can feel especially restrictive in your later years. If you experience pain due to lateral collateral ligament (LCL) and medial collateral ligament (MCL) injuries, you will have to exercise some caution. Regular sessions on your chair can help you keep your body fit and flexible, without stressing your knees.

Consult your doctor and discuss the depth of your injury. Keep your sessions short and only increase your intensity when you are comfortable and given permission by your physical therapist or doctor.

Asanas That Help Your Knees

Focus on gentle stretches. Using your chair, you can focus on proper form without worrying about balancing or aggravating your knee(s). If a movement causes any pain, do not continue. Always check your knee and leg after yoga practice for any swelling.

Seated flexing foot pose: Helps stretch your foot and leg gently, warming the area around your knee joint.

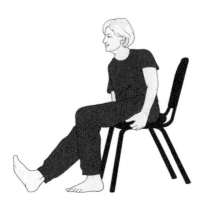

1. Stretch your leg to the front.
2. Point your toes toward you and hold for 30 seconds. Breathe.
3. Release. Repeat twice before switching to your other foot.

Chair stick pose: Allows your knee to be stretched safely.

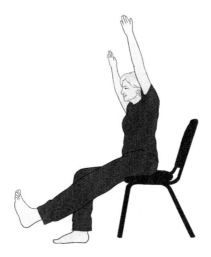

1. Raise your arms above your head.
2. Extend your right leg and lift your lower leg (from knee down) off the ground.
3. Flex your ankle, pointing the toes at you. Hold for two breaths.
4. Feel the stretch in your quads and hamstring.
5. Switch sides. Flow between left and right three times on each side.

Seated lunge: Stretches your thigh, hamstrings, and knee.

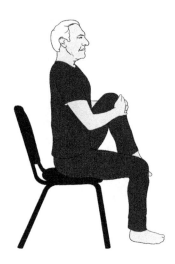

1. Keep the back straight and long in your seat.
2. Plant your left foot on the ground.
3. Inhale and grasp your hands around your right thigh to lift your right leg up.
4. Slowly pull your leg up and hug your knee to your chest.
5. Hold for two breaths and slowly release.
6. Repeat two more times and switch to the other leg.

YOGA FOR BACK PAIN

A stiff back with tight muscles and a limited range of motion can bring a sense of restriction. Back pain is a common injury, often from slips, falls, and repetitive strain. When the back is tight, it can create increasing problems with balance and cause even further limitations. Without being able to move freely, you may start to move less, and your pain may increase. Chair yoga can help you feel relief from tight muscles by stretching and improving both your circulation and range of motion, reducing the risk of arthritis. If you have spinal injuries or chronic pain, consult your doctor before practicing.

Asanas for Back Pain

Know your limitations before practicing and avoid trying to do too much too soon. Regular deep breathing will help you increase your circulation and relieve tension that you may carry in your back.

Cat-cow flow in chair: Opens your chest area and stretches your upper and lower back.

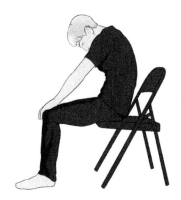

1. Inhale. Slowly push your chest out as you take your shoulders back (cow pose).
2. Exhale. Bring your chest, shoulders, and face into your body, dropping your chin toward the chest (cat pose).
3. Repeat the flow of cow to cat, following your breath, for four rounds.

Cobra in chair: Engages your upper and mid back while opening your chest.

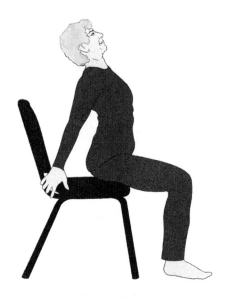

1. Reach behind to grasp the chair behind you.
2. Inhale and lift your chest and lower the shoulders, looking up to the ceiling.
3. Exhale as you hold the stretch, head tilted back.

4. Hold for six breaths.

5. Release. Repeat for one more round of six breaths.

Seated folded pose with bolster variation: Allows your lower back muscles to stretch and relax.

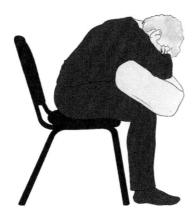

1. Take your bolster or pillow and place it atop your thighs.

2. Inhale and lift your arms overhead.

3. As you exhale, extend your arms forward and lower your torso slowly onto the bolster. Your torso will come to rest on the bolster as you reach for the ground. Go only as far as comfortable.

4. Hold for four breaths.

5. Release and slowly lift up. Rest and repeat for four more breaths.

POST-SURGERY YOGA

Surgery can limit your ability to practice and exercise, but you can still slowly build your stamina and mobility. Before and after your surgery can be times to engage in exercise to help prepare your body and help it heal. Gentle exercise can help reduce the risk of any post-surgery injuries developing and helps improve your mood and mindset.

Use caution and always speak to your surgeon before engaging in any physical activity. If you feel pain or discomfort, stop.

Post-surgery Asanas to Help Heal

Post-operation can involve time in bed or a chair, resting and recuperating from injury. When you have the okay from your doctor, you can try some asanas that can help you feel more energy and relaxation.

Seated palms on belly: Grounds you and focuses on the breath.

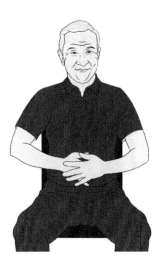

1. Sit grounded with your feet firmly on the floor. All your toes and your heels should touch the ground.
2. Allow your back to lengthen, extending your shoulders, chest, and chin so that you sit tall.
3. Close your eyes and bring your hands to your navel.
4. Take deep breaths and long exhalations for six breaths.

Chair side bend: Improves breathing and brings lightness to the ribcage, hips, and belly.

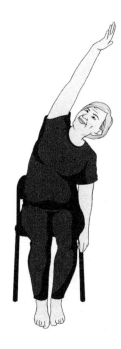

1. Hold the chair with your left hand.
2. Inhale as you raise your right arm out to the side until you are pointing at the ceiling.
3. Exhale and feel the stretch on your right side.
4. Slowly inhale as you extend your arm over your head, reaching to the left for a slight bend.
5. Hold for six breaths and release, bringing your arm back.
6. Repeat twice and switch to the left side.

Seated pelvic tilt and tuck: Engages your core muscles and supports the hips and pelvic area)

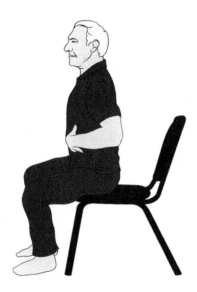

1. Inhale as you lift your chest upward, engaging your upper abdomen. Let your spine lengthen upward so that your tailbone moves out, causing a slight arch in your spine.
2. Exhale and inhale three times.
3. Exhale and release. Your chest and abdomen will return to a centered position as your tailbone comes inward.
4. Repeat six times.

STROKE RECOVERY YOGA

Yoga's benefits for the mind-body connection can help the recovery of stroke sufferers by engaging the mind and body to work together. Balance and gait are frequent problems for stroke patients, who may experience decreased mobility due to the fear of falling and loss of stamina. Using breathing, awareness, and asanas, you can help rewire your brain to improve movement and functionality.

Include a guided meditation in your yoga practice, for 5 to 10 minutes, to help engage the mind and bring awareness to your body.

Asanas for Stroke Recovery

Using a chair will help you feel grounded and safe during your practice. Even with small movements, continue to breathe to maximize the benefits. Consult your doctor and follow any guidelines you are given. At any point, you can stop and find your balance again, and only go within your own limitations.

Neck rolls: Eases tension in the neck and reconnects your breath to your movements.

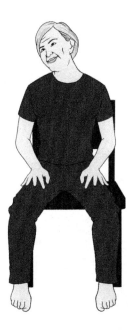

1. From the center, exhale as you slowly take your neck down toward the right shoulder.
2. Hold for two breaths. Release and inhale as you lift your neck and head to center again.
3. Repeat on the left side for two breaths.
4. Complete four rounds of this movement.

Seated hip circles: Rebuilds balance and mobility in your hip and pelvic area.

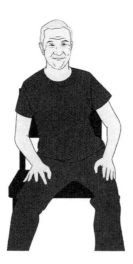

1. Lengthen your spine and place your hands on the thighs.
2. Slowly, begin to circle your torso at the hips.
3. Inhale as you push your torso forward.
4. Exhale as you circle your torso back.
5. Return to center.
6. Repeat in the other direction.

Modified eagle arms: Engages your mind as you focus on relaxing your upper body and hands.

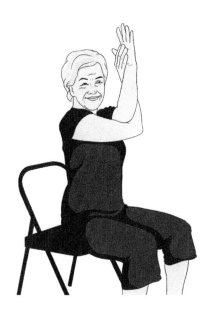

1. Inhale and extend your arms forward at shoulder level.
2. Cross your left arm over your right and bend your elbows.
3. Bring your bent arms toward your chest as you press your forearms together.
4. If able, press the palms together.
5. Hold for three deep breaths.
6. Release by unfolding your arms.
7. Repeat by crossing your right arm over your left arm.

YOGA FOR TRAUMA RECOVERY AND HIGH-STRESS

The restorative aspects of yoga can help relieve trauma. The eight limbs of yoga can help relieve anxiety and stress when used together. As Bessel Van Der Kolk wrote in *The Body Keeps the Score*, yoga can help manage and reduce the effects of trauma both in the mind and in the body (van der Kolk, 2015). No matter your past or present, yoga can be there for you.

Asanas for Trauma Recovery and High-Stress

Practice asanas with meditation and go slowly. If you start to feel overwhelmed, stop until you can ground yourself and get regulated. You can stop for the day and decide to go even slower next time. It's not a race, and you want your yoga and meditation practice to be a safe place for you. Consult with your doctor and therapist to understand any concerns you may have.

Hands to heart: Brings more awareness to your breath and grounds you.

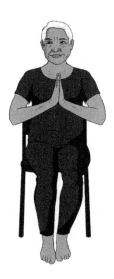

1. Sit in your chair and inhale slowly through your nose as you keep your arms relaxed.
2. Exhale and raise your hands in a prayer position to your chest.
3. Rest your thumbs gently against your heart area.
4. Inhale again through the nose and notice how it feels as it fills your lungs. Notice the energy flowing through your body. Let it out in a long exhale.
5. Continue to breathe, observing how your body feels physically as you follow the breath.

6. Inhale and exhale for 12 rounds before releasing and placing your hands in your lap.

Chair raised hands pose—Urdhva Hastasana: Brings an energizing stretch to your upper body.

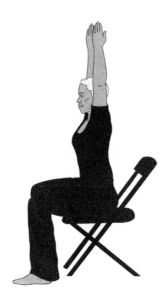

1. Inhale and place your hands on your thighs.
2. Exhale as you lift your arms to the sky, following the movement with your eyes until your chin lifts.
3. Hold for three breaths before putting your arms down and sitting up straight.

Chair warrior pose I and II: Engages many muscles in your torso and legs and revitalizes your mind.

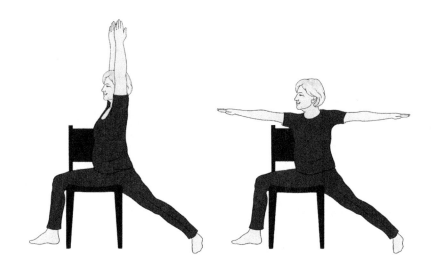

1. In the chair, inhale as you bring your left foot out to the side, pointing your toes out with your knee bent.
2. Extend your right foot behind you to the right of your chair.
3. Exhale and bring your arms up to shoulder level. Look out over your left hand.
4. Inhale and exhale deeply, holding for three breaths.
5. Inhale to release and return to center.
6. Repeat on the other side, bending your right knee and extending the left leg behind. Hold for three breaths.

YOGA FOR HIGH BLOOD PRESSURE

A study from the Center for Disease Control shows that 1 in 3 Americans have high blood pressure, which is also called hypertension. This condition can be caused by stress and lack of physical activity, increasing the risk of heart disease and stroke. In addition to your medication and dietary changes, adding yoga to your weekly routine can help you with weight loss, stress reduction, and increased physical fitness (Stelter, 2018).

Asanas for High Blood Pressure

When diagnosed with high blood pressure, consult with your doctor for any underlying conditions and be mindful of any instructions. Specific yoga asanas, such as backward bends and inversions (with the heart higher than the head), should be avoided. With chair yoga, you can focus on what feels good for your body and will help you internally as well.

Chair pigeon pose: Stretches and mobilizes your legs, hips, and pelvis.

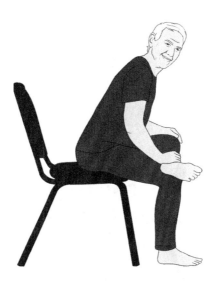

1. Inhale and hold your right thigh in your hands as you raise your right leg.
2. Place your right leg over your left thigh.
3. When comfortable, sit straight.
4. Take two deep breaths and release.
5. Repeat on the left side for two breaths.
6. Repeat twice more on each side.

Chair twist: Allows your abdomen and hips to work in sync with your torso and back, massaging the inner organs.

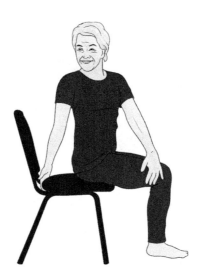

1. Inhale and lengthen your spine as you roll your shoulders back and down.
2. Keep your core muscles engaged as you exhale.
3. Gently twist your torso to the right, moving from the belly button upward. Keep your pelvis and knees facing forward.
4. Grasp the back of the chair to hold for two rounds of breathing.
5. Release as you exhale, coming back to center.
6. Repeat to the left.
7. Twist each side five times.

Chair Savasana (corpse pose): Brings your mind and body to a state of relaxation and calm.

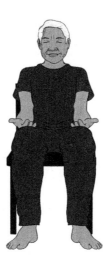

1. You can use this pose on a chair or bed. It is good to end each yoga practice with Savasana.
2. In a chair, sit with your eyes closed and your hands resting loosely in your lap.
3. Let your spine remain long and the shoulders back.
4. Observe any sensations in your body.
5. Start with 12 rounds of breathing. You can sit in Savasana for as long as needed.

YOGA FOR JOINT, ARTHRITIC, OR RHEUMATIC PAIN

Discomfort caused by the joints, arthritis, and rheumatic pain can interfere with your daily routine. Avoiding exercise can make those problems even worse. Chair yoga is an effective treatment that can ease symptoms.

Asanas for Joint, Arthritic, or Rheumatic Pain

When it comes to pain in your joints and flare-ups in arthritis, do what you can. Avoid stressing your body to try to do a pose you aren't ready for. Keep your movements slow and flowing to get the maximum benefit.

Chair stick pose: Activates your quads while engaging your entire leg.

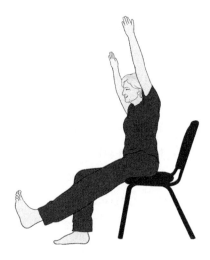

1. In a seated position, lift your right calf by extending your knee.
2. Lift only as high as you can.
3. Flex the right foot so your toes come toward you, pressing out with your heel.
4. Hold for two breaths.
5. Release and switch sides.
6. Repeat three times on each side.

Shoulder rolls and hand stretch: Lets your shoulders relieve tension and increases blood circulation to the arms and hands.

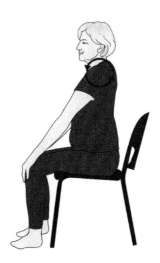

1. Inhale and begin to roll the shoulders, five full rotations in each direction.

2. Roll your wrists next, five times in each direction.
3. Open your hands and close them slowly. Repeat once.
4. Extend the right arm in front of you and turn your palm to face out in a "stop" pose.
5. With your left hand, place your palm over the right palm with the fingers pointed down. Your fingers on both hands should touch the opposite hand's wrist.
6. Hold for five breaths, release, and repeat on the other hand.
7. Shake it off.

Hands on knees: Relaxes your back and shoulders and massages your digestive system.

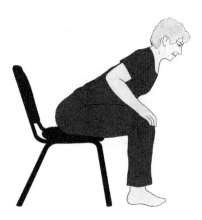

1. Inhale and extend your spine up.
2. Exhale as you bend forward slowly until your torso comes to 60 degrees, or as far as you're able.
3. Inhale as you lengthen your spine. Imagine someone gently pulling your torso forward but don't move your hips.
4. Exhale and look up. Remain here for six breaths.
5. Inhale as you release and come back to center.

YOGA FOR BALANCE OR INNER EAR PROBLEMS

Issues with balance, whether from muscle weakness or inner ear problems, can be a common reason why standing or moving fluidly is intimidating for new yoga practitioners. Using a chair can help you conquer the fear of falling, giving you a safe place to sit and exercise.

Asanas for Balance

If you are experiencing problems with your balance, check with your doctor before performing any asanas. Though a chair is a safer option than standing, you will want to be able to do the poses to the best of your ability. If closing your eyes or moving too quickly impairs your balance, move slower and keep your eyes open.

Chair mountain pose: Grounds you and warms up your body.

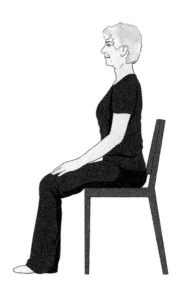

1. Inhale deeply and lengthen your back. Pull your shoulders back gently.
2. Exhale as you push down on your sit bones. Keep your knees bent and your feet on the floor.
3. Inhale deeply, exhale, and roll your shoulders again, taking them down and back.
4. Gently tighten your core muscles and keep your arms relaxed.
5. Hold for one minute of breathing.

Reverse arm hold: Opens your chest and deepens your breathing.

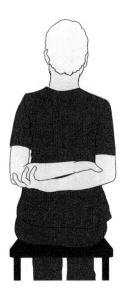

1. Inhale. Stretch both arms to the sides with your palms facing the floor.
2. Exhale and roll your shoulders forward. Let the hands swing behind your back.
3. Clasp your hands over their opposite elbow. Your left hand will grasp the right elbow, right hand grasps the left elbow.
4. Pull gently.
5. Hold for five breaths.
6. Release and switch your arms so that the one that had rested on top is now on the bottom. Hold for five breaths.

Chair cactus arms: Connects your upper body to the torso.

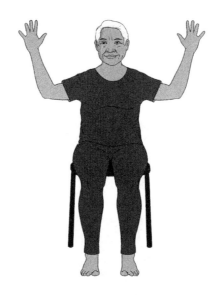

1. Inhale and raise your arms to shoulder level at your sides.
2. Exhale. Bend the elbows, feeling a stretch in the chest and shoulders.
3. Inhale. Open your arms wide, letting the chest expand. Keep your gaze focused ahead.
4. Hold for three breaths.
5. Inhale and release, bringing the arms down to your lap.
6. Repeat twice more.

YOGA IS ACCESSIBLE FOR ALL

When you see photos online of perfect poses that seem impossible, yoga can feel intimidating. If you have an illness or ailment that affects your ability to move easily or without pain, the thought of trying to achieve perfection can be overwhelming so you avoid it. But yoga isn't meant for just one body type. It can help many people, young or old, achieve better living.

The symptoms of major ailments, such as chronic pain or neurological limitations, need to be acknowledged but remember that with yoga, there is no rush or time limit. Practice within your own best abilities, giving yourself lots of rest as needed and modifying poses safely. Chair yoga can help you find the benefits of asanas and pranayama, without the worry of being able to stand or balance for long periods of time.

If you need to modify how long you hold a pose and how long you rest between each pose, that is still going to be beneficial. Allow your body to tell you when you need to rest and when you need to modify a pose. Stay mindful and your practice will continue to develop.

CONCLUSION

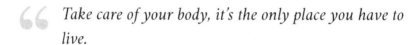 *Take care of your body, it's the only place you have to live.*

— JIM ROHN

The journey of yoga never ends. Just when you think you have learned something and can't learn anymore, you will discover something new about the practice. It may be a different asana that feels amazing or a new guided meditation that changes how you think. This continual sense of growth can keep yoga exciting and fun.

You've now learned the aspects of chair yoga and the principles that guide it. If you had experience, you had these concepts reiterated so that your mind can fully absorb and process them. No matter where you are in your practice, the act of learning can help your brain stay motivated and energized. In a 2013 study, seniors who learn a new skill have improved memory which helps improve cognition and retention (Quilian, 2016).

Chair yoga combines multiple skills and concepts within itself. Once you've started down the yogic path, there are many benefits for you. Even for those who are mobile but must sit at a desk throughout the day as part of their job, chair yoga has a number of benefits to keep the mind and body engaged. Through meditation and mindfulness, you will gain more control and awareness of your emotions, moods, and thoughts. Mindfulness combined with asanas will allow you to feel better physically and be able to participate more actively in daily life.

The long history of yoga gives you the knowledge you need to succeed. In a way, you are walking with the memories of millions of people over the course of history who have found yoga. In 2022, a survey estimated that over 34.3 million people in the United States now practice yoga regularly (Smith, 2022). The eight limbs of yoga can guide you along this path, giving you an awareness of the discipline and compassion that comes from yoga. Yoga as a way of life improves your inner and outer self and also gives you a sense of community. There are many online groups available to all levels of practitioners, and you can find a local group for extra support and to share in your journey.

The mind and body connection remains at the heart of yoga. With consistent meditation, you can bring a sense of calm to your asana practice and to your daily life. The asanas you've learned and practiced can ease tension and soreness while allowing your muscles to strengthen and your balance to improve. When you feel like you want to truly connect the mind and body, to feel mental clarity, practice the mudras that best suit your needs.

Though many people would recognize yoga by the asanas often portrayed in the media, you'll have learned how they can be modified and changed to suit your own body's needs. Chair yoga is meant to be accessible. Modifying asanas through tools can help make them achievable and improve your form. If you have a specific health concern, or develop one in the future, you can refer to Chapter 10 to help you modify your yoga practice safely.

The more consistently you practice, the more benefits you will find. The two-week program included is an example of how consistency, even for just a few days a week, can improve your mind and body in a short amount of time.

SHARE YOUR JOURNEY

You never know who could be helped by starting a yoga practice. It can be someone you love or someone you have never met before, across the country or the world. You can personally help one person, right now, in 2 minutes or less by going to Amazon and posting a review of this book. That one person, who needs this book and its teachings, will discover it through your review and learn what you have learned. Sharing the message of yoga can mean that you embody the spirit of generosity and service to others. Even if you don't consider yourself the type of person who usually leaves reviews, you can help someone else, instantly, by reviewing your order of this book on Amazon. I read every word, and your thoughts are so precious and valuable to me.

An example of how quickly yoga can change your life is Christine's story. Christine, a newer yoga practitioner, discovered the life-changing practice of yoga after an accident. After suffering from severe neck and shoulder pain and headaches, she decided to try yoga for just a week. That week changed her life when she began to feel better. Soon she was practicing regularly with little pain and the world around her seemed brighter and happier. She believed in herself and set the intention that she would take care of herself through yoga. Now she is a major supporter of yoga and what it can bring to others.

Listen to your body when it tells you when to change, when to challenge yourself, and when to rest. Some days you may sit in a chair to meditate and that is all you want to do. Other days you may want to move your body and really feel the strength and balance you've developed. Remember that chair yoga is a practice, and each practice may be different. Your goal is to keep practicing.

The most important thing for any yogi, of any ability, is to realize that the connection of mind, body, and spirit is essential to you and your health. Those three aspects come together through meditation, physical alignment, and mindfulness. As they do, your yoga practice will continue to improve and enrich your life for many years to come.

As Eleanor Roosevelt said, "Life was meant to be lived, and curiosity must be kept alive" (*Eleanor Roosevelt quotes*, n.d.). Start with your practice now and continue to stay curious and learning so that practicing becomes a joy. You will soon see that a simple beginning becomes the start of a beautiful journey that brings you health and happiness for many years to come.

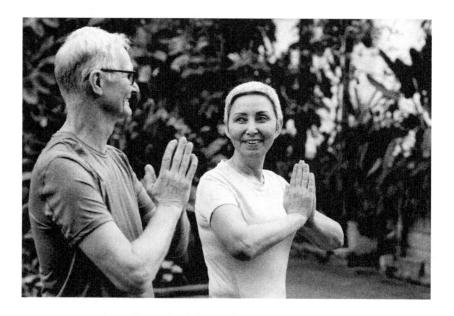

BONUS AUDIO MEDITATION

As a gift for you, I have recorded an exercise in *progressive muscle relaxation*, as featured in Chapter 5, to ease aches and pains and reduce stress and anxiety.

You can receive the free meditation by visiting

https://chapshawpublications.com/meditation

I hope you enjoy the meditation!

A QUICK NOTE

To post a review on Amazon, scan the code on the next page, or alternatively, find the book's page on Amazon and scroll down and click on "Write a customer review". You can also find this by going into "Orders" and clicking "Write a product review."

Then, you can enter in your thoughts and something you learned and click submit. You can even upload a photo of the book if you have it. Thank you so much! I really appreciate it!

If you would like to scan this code, open the camera on your phone and click on the link that comes up, or use a QR reader.

Overall rating

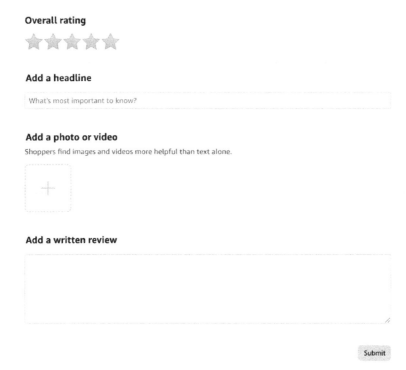

Add a headline

What's most important to know?

Add a photo or video

Shoppers find images and videos more helpful than text alone.

Add a written review

Submit

Screenshots retrieved from Amazon.com

REFERENCES

Arm stretches: For flexibility. (2016, May 12). Healthline. https://www.healthline.com/health/fitness-exercise/arm-stretches

Arthritis-related statistics. (2019). Centers for Disease Control and Prevention. https://www.cdc.gov/arthritis/data_statistics/arthritis-related-stats.htm

Ashish. (2020, March 17). *What are bandhas: Types, importance in yoga & benefits.* Fitsri. https://www.fitsri.com/yoga/bandhas

Ashish. (2021, October 27). *Samadhi explained: Its four stages and how to achieve it?* Fitsri. https://www.fitsri.com/articles/samadhi

Ashtanga (Eight limbs of yoga). (2020, October 3). In *Wikipedia.* https://en.wikipedia.org/wiki/Ashtanga_(eight_limbs_of_yoga)

Atkinson, A. (2016, October 21). *Chair yoga for stroke survivors* [Video]. YouTube. https://www.youtube.com/watch?v=89wkSAJYKEU

Bhandari, A. (2019, November 7). *B.K.S. Iyengar.* YogTravel. https://www.yogtravel.com/blog/bks-iyengar

Blick, K. (2017, December 14). *Combat the health risks that come with prolonged sitting by using these simple but effective seated yoga poses and stretches.* Allina Health.https://www.allinahealth.org/healthysetgo/move/energize-your-workday-with-upperbody-chair-yoga

Boland, K. (2019, June 1). *A chair yoga sequence for arthritis: Increase mobility and decrease pain.* YogaUOnline. https://www.yogauonline.com/yoga-for-arthritis/chair-yoga-sequence-for-arthritis-increase-mobility-and-decrease-pain

Bowie, D. (n.d.). *David Bowie quotes.* Goodreads. https://www.goodreads.com/quotes/9630789-aging-is-an-extraordinary-process-whereby-you-become-the-person

Brennan, D. (2021, October 25). *Benefits of yoga for mental health.* WebMD. https://www.webmd.com/balance/benefits-of-yoga-for-mental-health

A brief history of yoga. (2021, March 4). The Yoga Institute. https://theyogainstitute.org/a-brief-history-of-yoga

Burgin, T. (2014, April 14). *History of yoga.* Yoga Basics. https://www.yogabasics.com/learn/history-of-yoga

Burgin, T. (2015, November 11). *The five yamas of yoga.* Yoga Basics. https://www.yogabasics.com/learn/the-five-yamas-of-yoga

Burke, A. (n.d.). *Yoga and osteoporosis: the do's and don'ts.* Yoga International. https://yogainternational.com/article/view/yoga-and-osteoporosis-the-dos-and-donts

Burkhart, L. (2019, August 8). *Shoulder and neck chair yoga that you can do anywhere, anytime.* Wysefit. https://wysefit.com/blog/shoulder-and-neck-chair-yoga-that-you-can-do-anywhere-anytime

Callahan, A. (2018, October 2). *Yoga after an injury: Is it safe?* Wilmington Yoga. https://wilmingtonyogacenter.com/yoga-after-an-injury-is-it-safe

Carrico, M. (2021, March 23). *Get to know the 8 limbs of yoga.* Yoga Journal. https://www.yogajournal.com/yoga-101/philosophy/8-limbs-of-yoga/eight-limbs-of-yoga

Chair Surya Namaskar: Chair sun salutation. (n.d.). Tummee. https://www.tummee.com/yoga-sequences/chair-surya-namaskar-yoga-sequence

Chair yoga for senior citizens: Chair yoga for back pain. (n.d.). Tummee. https://www.tummee.com/yoga-sequences/senior-chair-yoga-back-pain

Chair yoga for seniors: Reduce pain and improve health [Video]. (n.d.). DailyCaring. https://dailycaring.com/chair-yoga-for-seniors-reduce-pain-and-improve-health-video

Cherry, K. (2022, September 8). *How meditation impacts your mind and body.* Verywell Mind. https://www.verywellmind.com/what-is-meditation-2795927#toc-impact-of-meditation

Chung, B. (2012, August 31). *The many uses of a yoga block.* DoYou. https://www.doyou.com/the-many-uses-of-a-yoga-block

Denslow, E. (Ed.). (2021, February 2). *5 huge benefits of yoga for stroke patients (& how to get started).* Flint Rehab. https://www.flintrehab.com/yoga-for-stroke-patients

DePaul, K. (2021, February 2). *What does it really take to build a new habit?* Harvard Business Review. https://hbr.org/2021/02/what-does-it-really-take-to-build-a-new-habit

Dowd-Higgins, C. (n.d.). *Be more mindful: 7 tips to improve your awareness.* Ellevate Network. https://www.ellevatenetwork.com/articles/6170-be-more-mindful-7-tips-to-improve-your-awareness

Eleanor Roosevelt quotes. (n.d.). BrainyQuote.com. Retrieved October 28, 2022, from BrainyQuote.com Web site: https://www.brainyquote.com/quotes/eleanor_roosevelt_126917

Elsey, E.L. (2013, June 28). *Relax your clients in under 5 minutes with these guided meditation scripts.* The Coaching Tools Company. https://www.thecoachingtoolscompany.com/de-stress-series-relax-clients-in-under-5-mins-guided-meditation-scripts

Exercise and stroke: How can exercise improve my health? (2013). The Stroke Association. https://www.stroke.org.uk/sites/default/files/exercise_and_stroke.pdf

Fascia Ball exercises. (n.d.). Blackroll. https://blackroll.com/exercises/product/fascia-ball-exercises

Ferdy, O. (2004, January 19). *One in five elderly have mobility problems.* CBS Netherlands. https://www.cbs.nl/en-gb/news/2004/04/one-in-five-elderly-have-mobility-problems

5 Surprising benefits of walking. (2019). Harvard Health. https://www.health.harvard.edu/staying-healthy/5-surprising-benefits-of-walking

Gill, B. (2017, June 22). *New to visualization? Here are 5 steps to get you started.* Forbes. https://www.forbes.com/sites/bhaligill/2017/06/22/new-to-visualization-here-are-5-steps-to-get-you-started

"The Good News" by Thich Nhat Hanh. (2015, December 3). Words for the Year. https://wordsfortheyear.com/2015/12/03/the-good-news-by-thich-nhat-hanh

Gumaer, D. (2021, February 18). *Weak legs in elderly adults: Causes, risks, home care.* Griswold Home Care. https://www.griswoldhomecare.com/blog/2021/february/weak-legs-in-elderly-adults-causes-risks-home-ca

Helfer, F. (2019, August 19). *How to use a yoga strap: 18 yoga strap stretches for beginners.* Yoga Rove. https://yogarove.com/yoga-strap-stretches-beginners

Heyman, J. (2019). *Accessible yoga: Poses and practices for every body.* Shambhala.

Hoien, E. (2020, May 6). *Self myofascial release techniques using massage balls.* Tune up Fitness. https://www.tuneupfitness.com/blog/self-myofascial-release-techniques-using-massage-balls

Hoogeboom, T. J., Dronkers, J. J., Hulzebos, E. H. J., & van Meeteren, N. L. U. (2014). *Merits of exercise therapy before and after major surgery.* Current Opinion in Anaesthesiology, 27(2), 161–166. https://doi.org/10.1097/aco.0000000000000062

How to do easy pose with neck stretch. (2015, April 12). Everyday Yoga. https://www.everydayyoga.com/blogs/guides/how-to-do-easy-pose-with-neck-stretch

How to meditate. (2020, February 26). Mindful. https://www.mindful.org/how-to-meditate

How to use a massage ball. (2020, April 14). The Physio Company. https://thephysiocompany.co.uk/how-to-use-a-massage-ball

How to use a yoga bolster. (n.d.). Everyday Yoga. https://www.everydayyoga.com/blogs/official/how-to-use-a-yoga-bolster

Hullett, A. (2020, August 27). *Take a seat: 11 chair yoga poses to try.* Greatist. https://greatist.com/move/chair-yoga

Iyengar, B. K. S. (2019). *Light on life: The yoga journey to wholeness, inner peace and ultimate freedom.* Hodder & Stoughton General Division.

Jain, R. (2019, June 13). *What are the 7 chakras? A guide of the energy centers and their effects.* Arhanta Yoga Ashram. https://www.arhantayoga.org/blog/7-chakras-introduction-energy-centers-effect

Joint freeing series (JFS): A beginner level practice to increase the mobility of joints. (n.d.). Tummee. https://www.tummee.com/yoga-sequences/beginner-joint-freeing-series

Julien. (2022, April 6). *The best yoga chairs, what are they and how to use them properly.* The Yoga Nomads. https://www.theyoganomads.com/yoga-chair

Larkin, B. (2021, July 20). *What is asteya? 5 powerful ways to practice non-stealing in yoga and life.* Brett Larkin. https://www.brettlarkin.com/what-is-asteya

Life force seal. (2017, March 8). Yoga Journal. https://www.yogajournal.com/practice/energetics/mudra/prana-mudra

Lin, H. (2021, July 8). *Where is the torso located on the body?*Reference.com. https://www.reference.com/science/torso-located-body-db3b4c3d89ceeaa2

Lindberg, S. (2020, August 24). *What are chakras? Meaning, location, and how to unblock them.* Healthline. https://www.healthline.com/health/what-are-chakras

Lutz, J. (2018, July 10). *Chair yoga: Gentle, effective exercise for osteoarthritis pain.* Practical Pain Management. https://patient.practicalpainmanagement.com/treatments/alternative/chair-yoga-gentle-effective-exercise-osteoarthritis-pain

Marchese, G. (2021, April 10). *8 Yoga poses to soothe neck pain & tension.*Yoga

Journal. https://www.yogajournal.com/poses/anatomy/neck/8-yoga-poses-to-soothe-neck-tension

Martins, F. (2021, February 28). *Chair yoga precautions.* Aura Wellness Center. https://aurawellnesscenter.com/2021/02/28/chair-yoga-precautions

Mayo Clinic Staff. (2018). *Sciatica-symptoms and causes.* Mayo Clinic. https://www.mayoclinic.org/diseases-conditions/sciatica/symptoms-causes/syc-20377435

Mayo Clinic Staff. (2020, August 1). *Frozen shoulder-symptoms and causes.* Mayo Clinic. https://www.mayoclinic.org/diseases-conditions/frozen-shoulder/symptoms-causes/syc-20372684

MD(Ayu), D. J. V. H. (2020, April 24). *Adi mudra–meaning, method of doing, benefits, dosha effect.* Easy Ayurveda. https://www.easyayurveda.com/2020/04/24/adi-mudra

Metivier, A. (2020, October 23). *Magnetic memory method-memory improvement made easy with Anthony Metivier.* Magnetic Memory Method-How to Memorize with a Memory Palace. https://www.magneticmemorymethod.com/how-to-visualize-clearly

Mike, G. (2021, December 9). *Yoga eye pillows and what they can do for you.* Yogigo. https://yogigo.com/yoga-eye-pillow-benefits

Mindfulness exercises. (2020, September 15). Mayo Clinic. https://www.mayoclinic.org/healthy-lifestyle/consumer-health/in-depth/mindfulness-exercises/art-20046356

Misiak, A. (n.d.). *Why we practice: A short history of yoga in the west.* Yoga International. https://yogainternational.com/article/view/why-we-practice-a-short-history-of-yoga-in-the-west/

More evidence that exercise can boost mood. (2019, May). Harvard Health. https://www.health.harvard.edu/mind-and-mood/more-evidence-that-exercise-can-boost-mood

Naskar, A. (2021, November 23). *9 best yoga chairs for great support and flexibility.* STYLECRAZE. https://www.stylecraze.com/articles/best-yoga-chair

Nhat Hanh, T. (1996, January 1). *Call me by my true names: The collected poems of Thich Nhat Hanh.* Parallax Press.

9 benefits of yoga. (2021). John Hopkins Medicine. https://www.hopkinsmedicine.org/health/wellness-and-prevention/9-benefits-of-yoga

Parsloe, Y. (2022, January 27). *What is chair yoga?* Yoga Pose. https://yogapose.com/articles/what-is-chair-yoga/

Pelzer, K. (2021, September 24). *Take a deep breath in, now release, and find inner peace with these 100 yoga quotes!* Parade. https://parade.com/1158471/kelseypelzer/yoga-quotes/

Piparaiya, N. (2020, December 10). *Activating the joints with Yogic Sukshma Vyayama.* Yoga U Online. https://www.yogauonline.com/yoga-basics/acti vating-joints-yogic-sukshma-vyayama

Pizer, A. (2020, February 26). *10 yoga poses you can do in a chair.* Verywell Fit. https://www.verywellfit.com/chair-yoga-poses-3567189

Plantar Fasciitis-symptoms and causes. (2018). Mayo Clinic. https://www.mayoclinic.org/diseases-conditions/plantar-fasciitis/symptoms-causes/syc-20354846

Powell, L. (2020, December 1). *13 key tips for creating a successful yoga lifestyle.* Yoga Basics. https://www.yogabasics.com/explore/yogic-lifestyle/yoga-lifestyle-tips

Quilian, C. (2016, August 31). *The importance of learning something new as you age.* Metro Health Inc. https://metrohealthinc.com/2016/08/31/the-importance-of-learning-something-new-as-you-age

Ransom, L. A. R., & Story, S. (2016, June 28). *Healing chair yoga: Shoulders.* Anjali Yoga Room. http://anjaliyogaroom.com/healing-chair-yoga-shoulders

Remski, M. (2017, April 12). *10 things we didn't know about yoga until this new must-read dropped.* Yoga Journal. https://www.yogajournal.com/yoga-101/history-of-yoga/10-things-didnt-know-yoga-history

Rogers, P. (2018). *How can you exercise and stretch the hamstring muscles?* Verywell Fit. https://www.verywellfit.com/hamstring-muscle-anatomy-and-stretches-3498372

Roosevelt, E. (2018). *The autobiography of Eleanor Roosevelt.* Zed.

Sander, S. (2017, December 29). *Yoga poses: warrior I, warrior II, and warrior III (Virabhadrasana).* Z Living. https://www.zliving.com/fitness/yoga/warrior-i-warrior-ii-warrior-iii-virabhadasana-tips-benefits-follow-up-poses-94452

Savage, J. (2020, June 12). *Chair yoga sequence for hips and hamstrings.* Ekhart Yoga. https://www.ekhartyoga.com/articles/practice/chair-yoga-sequence-hips-and-hamstrings

Schware, R. (2013, May 13). *A call to service: Sharing yoga as a tool of self-empow-erment.* HuffPost. https://www.huffpost.com/entry/yoga-self-empowerment_b_3141147

Seated cat cow pose. (n.d.). Yogapedia.com. https://www.yogapedia.com/yoga-poses/seated-cat-cow-pose/11/11583

Seladi-Schulman, J. (2018, August 27). *Arm.* Healthline Media. https://www.healthline.com/human-body-maps/arm

Selig, M. (2018). *6 ways to discover and choose your core values.* Psychology Today. https://www.psychologytoday.com/us/blog/changepower/201811/6-ways-discover-and-choose-your-core-values

Seniors yoga sequence: Chair yoga sequence for seniors. (n.d.). Tummee. https://www.tummee.com/yoga-sequences/yoga-sequence-for-seniors-restorative-and-chair-poses

Smith, L. (2022, October 7). *41 yoga statistics: How many people practice yoga?* The Good Body. https://www.thegoodbody.com/yoga-statistics

Stelter, G. (2015, December 7). *Chair yoga for seniors: Seated poses.* Healthline. https://www.healthline.com/health/fitness-exercise/chair-yoga-for-seniors

Stelter, G. (2018, March 2). *Yoga for high blood pressure: A gentle routine.* Healthline. https://www.healthline.com/health/fitness-exercise/yoga-for-high-blood-pressure

Stevens, T. (2014, August 1). *Chair yoga exercises for the feet and toes.* Little Flower Yoga. https://www.littlefloweryoga.com/blog/chair-yoga-exercises-for-the-feet-and-toes

Stiles, R. (2022, February 22). *6 yoga poses for high blood pressure.* Yoga Journal. https://www.yogajournal.com/poses/yoga-by-benefit/high-blood-pressure/yoga-for-high-blood-pressure

Symptoms of blocked chakras. (2020, September 6). Yoga Signs. https://yogasigns.com/symptoms-of-blocked-chakras

Taylor, Dr. M. J. (2015, June 17). *THe power and science of mudra.* Smart Safe Yoga. https://smartsafeyoga.com/the-power-and-science-of-mudra

The power of yoga mudras to awaken the five elements. (2020, July 6). TINT Yoga. https://tintyoga.com/magazine/yoga-mudra

Tomlinson, K. (2016, April 14). *An introduction to mudras.* Ekhart Yoga. https://www.ekhartyoga.com/articles/practice/an-introduction-to-mudras

Torres, M. (2020, October 9). *Knee pain yoga exercises.* KneeForce. https://kneeforce.com/knee-pain-yoga-exercises

Trauma sensitive yoga sequence: Yoga for trauma survivors with restorative yoga

sequence. (n.d.). Tummee. https://www.tummee.com/yoga-sequences/trauma-sensitive-yoga-sequence

van der Kolk, B. (2015). *The body keeps the score: Mind, Brain and body in the transformation of trauma.* Penguin Books.

Walters, O. (2022, March 7). *Importance of core strength: 11 benefits of a strong core.* Healthline. https://www.healthline.com/health/core-strength-more-important-than-muscular-arms

What is causing my neck pain and headache? (2021, November 9). Healthline. https://www.healthline.com/health/stiff-neck-and-headache

What is shunya mudra? (2018, August 27). Yogapedia.com. https://www.yogapedia.com/definition/6859/shunya-mudra

What is surya mudra? (2017, July 26). Yogapedia.com. https://www.yogapedia.com/definition/6869/surya-mudra

Yoga and high blood pressure. (2022, May 1). Harvard Health. https://www.health.harvard.edu/heart-health/yoga-and-high-blood-pressure

Yoga for all: Himalayan yoga tradition - joints and glands exercises. (n.d.). Tummee. https://www.tummee.com/yoga-sequences/himalayan-tradition-yoga-sequence-joints-glands

Yoga for neck pain: 12 poses to try. (2018, February 15). Healthline. https://www.healthline.com/health/yoga-for-neck-pain

Yoga for the immune system: Therapy yoga for those with immunodeficiency. (n.d.). Tummee. https://www.tummee.com/yoga-sequences/immune-system-yoga-sequence

Yoga modifications after a knee injury. (2021, February 27). Body by Yoga. https://bodybyyoga.training/yoga-for-beginners/modifications/yoga-modifications-after-a-knee-injury/

Yoga success stories! (2014, July 3). The Yoga Room. https://www.rryogaroom.com/the-yoga-room/yoga-success-stories-2

Yoga: Common contraindications you should know. (2021, March 8). Fitpage. https://fitpage.in/yoga-common-contraindications-you-should-know

Yogi reveals 10 chair yoga moves for people with knee pain. (2020, June 8). Power of Positivity: Positive Thinking & Attitude. https://www.powerofpositivity.com/chair-yoga-seated-poses-for-knee-pain

Zakaria, N. (2021, September 15). *Ten yoga mudras and their benefits.* Dragonfly Yoga Studio. https://www.dragonfly-yoga.org/blog/ten-yoga-mudras-and-their-benefits-1#

IMAGE REFERENCES

Aurelius, M. (2021, February 11). *Couple smiling while looking at each other* [Image]. Pexels. https://www.pexels.com/photo/couple-smiling-while-looking-at-each-other-6787520

Franco, D. (2016, February 7). *Person's hand in shallow focus* [Image]. Unsplash. https://unsplash.com/photos/CeZypKDceQc

Gonullu, M. (2021, February 19) *Senior asian woman in striped sweater meditating* [Image]. Pexel. https://www.pexels.com/photo/senior-asian-woman-in-striped-sweatshirt-meditating-6888687

Kopřiva, J. (2021, January 25). *Man in black crew neck t-shirt sitting on black leather armchair* [Image]. Unsplash. https://unsplash.com/photos/FNA2fSVXKTo

Los Muertos Crew. (2021, March 25). *Elderly woman meditating* [Image]. Pexels. https://www.pexels.com/photo/elderly-woman-meditating-7260776

Makagonova, K. (2018, June 6). *Person doing meditation outdoors photo* [Image]. Unsplash. https://unsplash.com/photos/V-TIPBoC_2M

Nilov, M. (2021, April 13). *Elderly man doing yoga* [Image]. Pexels. https://www.pexels.com/photo/elderly-man-doing-yoga-7500645

Nilov, M. (2021, February 27). *A couple doing arm stretching* [Image]. Pexels. https://www.pexels.com/photo/a-couple-doing-arm-stretching-6975765

RODNAE Productions. (2021, June 11). *Photo of a kid playing with her grandfather* [Image]. Pexels. https://www.pexels.com/photo/photo-of-a-kid-playing-with-her-grandfather-8298446

RODNAE Productions. (2021, June 2). *An elderly woman in white tank top raising her hands* [Image]. Pexels. https://www.pexels.com/photo/an-elderly-woman-in-white-tank-top-raising-her-hands-8172936

ABOUT THE AUTHOR

Jeanne Chapshaw, yoga teacher, writer, educator, and health worker, created Chapshaw Publications to help seniors and those who work with them find joy, wellness, and movement through activities.

Experienced in teaching physical fitness, mindfulness and meditation to seniors and those of all ages, Jeanne and a deeply caring team of writers and researchers together are creating resources for seniors to enjoy the moment, find connection in their golden years, and embrace the time ahead. Each team member has personally loved seniors living in assist- ed living and has a passion for facilitating enjoyment no matter the age or ability.

The mission is to share quality information and provide exercises and activities that have been vetted by experts as safe, effective, and enjoy- able. While books cannot replace in-person experiences, the hope is that words in this book will transfer into health and peace that is accessible to anyone, at any time.

Chapshaw Publications is the brand behind Chair Yoga for Seniors Over 60 and Guided Wellness Journal for Self-Care, Fitness & Mindfulness.

If you have any questions or suggestions, we welcome feedback. Please send an email to

hello@chapshawpublications.com. Thank you for reading!